# Digital Babylon

## HOLLYWOOD, INDIEWOOD & DOGME 95

D1520790

shari roman

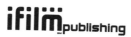
ifilm publishing

**DIGITAL BABYLON**
**Hollywood, Indiewood and Dogme 95**
Copyright © 2001 Shari Roman

LONE EAGLE PUBLISHING COMPANY, LLC™
1024 N. Orange Dr.
Hollywood, CA 90038
Phone 323.308.3400 or 800.815.0503
A division of IFILM® Corporation, www.ifilmpro.com

Printed in the United States of America
10 9 8 7 6 5 4 3 2 1

Cover design and creative direction by Sean Alatorre
Book design by Carla Green

Library of Congress Cataloging-in-Publication Data
Roman, Shari
    Digital Babylon : Hollywood, Indiewood & Dogme '95 / by Shari Roman ; with a foreword by Harmony Korine
        p.   cm.
    Includes indexes.
        1. Experimental films--History and criticism. 2. Independent filmmakers.
    3. Dogme 95 (Group) 4. Digital cinematography. I. Title.

    PN1995.9.E96 R58 2001
    791.43--dc21                                        2001038281

Books may be purchased in bulk at special discounts for promotional or educational purposes. Special editions can be created to specifications. Inquiries for sales and distribution, textbook adoption, foreign language translation, editorial, and rights and permissions inquiries should be addressed to: Jeff Black, IFILM Publishing, 1024 N. Orange Dr., Hollywood, CA 90038 or send e-mail to: info@ifilm.com

Distributed to the trade by National Book Network, 800-462-6420

IFILM® and Lone Eagle Publishing Company™ are registered trademarks.

Portions of some interviews in this book have previously appeared in *Flaunt* magazine, *Fade In* magazine, *The Face* (UK), *The Guardian* (UK), *Res* magazine and IFILM.com.

Jean-Luc Godard essay (1995), courtesy of the Montreal Film Festival, Daniele Cauchard, vice-president.

Wim Wenders essay, courtesy of the author.

Images from *The Celebration*, *julien donkey-boy* and *Mifune* by Anthony Dod Mantle.

Cover photo: Bjork in *Dancer in the Dark*, courtesy of Fine Line Features.

# CONTENTS

**ACKNOWLEDGMENTS** v

**PREFACE** vi

**FOREWORD** by Harmony Korine viii

**SECTION 1: PAST AND FUTURE**

JEAN-LUC GODARD:
THE FUTURE OF CINEMA 1

OLD WAVES, NEW INFLUENCES 4

PRODUCERS COMMENTARY 15
    JASON KLIOT 15
    PETER BRODERICK 22
    SCOTT MACAULAY 28

**SECTION 2: DOGME 95 AND THE NEW GUARD**

WIM WENDERS: WHAT THE
NEW TECHNOLOGIES OFFER 35

THE MANIFESTO 40

THE VOW OF CHASTITY 41

THE MEN WHO WOULD BE DOGME 42

10 INSIDER TIPS TO DOGME 95:
NARRATIVE, DIALOGUE, LOGISTICS 56

ORIGINAL DOGME 58
    HARMONY KORINE 58
    SØREN KRAGH-JACOBSEN 63
    The Confession of Søren Kragh-Jacobsen 67
    JEAN MARC BARR 68
    KRISTIAN LEVRING 71
    THOMAS VINTERBERG 79
    The Confession of Thomas Vinterberg 88
    LARS VON TRIER 89

DOGME FILMS TO DATE 97

LIGHTS, CAMERA, DIGITAL ACTION!          103
DPs AT WORK                              103
   MARYSE ALBERTI                        104
   JOHN BAILEY                           112
   ANTHONY DOD MANTLE                    128

SECTION 3:   **BEYOND DOGME**

MIKE FIGGIS: RISKING THE FUTURE          136

RIDING THE EDGE: DIRECTORS               141
   ALLISON ANDERS                        142
   JENNIFER JASON LEIGH
      & ALAN CUMMING                     145
   MIGUEL ARTETA                         152
   PETER GREENAWAY                       154
   JIM JARMUSCH                          161
   RICHARD LINKLATER                     165
   GUS VAN SANT                          171
   AGNES VARDA                           178
   WIM WENDERS                           182

DV, FILM FESTIVALS AND THE PRESS         189
   GEOFFREY GILMORE
   PIERS HANDLING                        196
   TODD MCCARTHY                         203

CRITICAL REVIEWS                         212
   VARIETY
   Deep Focus: At Cannes '98,
   Dogma 95 has its day                  212

   FILM COMMENT
   Straight to Film: Can video
   cut it on the big screen?             214

   PREMIERE
   Cinema Purité                         217

**REFERENCES AND RESOURCES**

A VERY BRIEF TECHNICAL GLOSSARY          223

GOING GLOBAL: DV TRANSFER HOUSES         225

RESOURCES AND WEBLINKS                   227

# ACKNOWLEDGMENTS

*Deepest Honors:* The existence of this book owes itself to Lars von Trier, Thomas Vinterberg, Søren Kragh-Jacobsen, Kristian Levring, Peter Aalbaek Jensen, Christel Hammer, everyone at *Nimbus Films, Zentropa Entertainments* and all the extraordinary individuals who gave their time and shared their knowledge for these interviews. You have been very generous to me.

*The Aces:* Todd McCarthy, who inspired me to go off to Copenhagen to interview von Trier for the short film which became *Lars from 1-10.* Sophie Fiennes, for her outstanding excellence in general, for our *Lars from 1-10* collaboration in particular and for showing me Billie Whitelaw in Beckett's *Not I.* John Pierson, who agreed to send us off to Copenhagen to interview Lars for his Independent Film Channel program, *Split Screen.* Anthony Dod Mantle, a genius DP and a stunning human being in all regards. Holly Willis, a book editor sublime. Lawrence Schubert, a brilliant editorial consultant, and *Flaunt* magazine who gave me a place to call home.

*Docents:* Carl Gottlieb, David Liu.

*My Europeans:* Marina Guinness, Laurence Miolano & Sandor Sagi, Margaux Murray, David & Lis Ponte, Maggie Swinfen, Damon Wise, for making space.

*Touchstones:* Steve Anderson, Iji Asfaw, Esther Bell, Luca Bercovici, Jeanne & Bob Berney, Angel Borrero, Ken Bowser & Susan Korda, Margot Breier, Richard Brown, Connie Conrad, Wendy Dembo, Alice Fisher, James Ferrera, Fifi, Anne Grossman, Trevor Groth, David Heyman, Steve Hochman, Jesper Jargil, Audrey Kelly, Lance Loud, Craig McLean, Thomas Mai, Nancy Main, Susan Mainzer, James Mathers, Conor McPherson, Richard Metzger, Marianne Meyer plus three, RJ Millard, the MRPM-ers, Steve Nalepa, Kavi Ohri & Teena Kang, RD Robb, Murray Roman, Douglas Rushkoff, Oberon Sinclair, Alexander Stuart & Charong Chow, Sharon Swart, Michael Tighe, Robin & Adam Turnier, for a whole bunch of site specific reasons.

*The IFILM Publishing Wizards:* Jeff Black, Carla Green, Lauren Rossini and Sean Alatorre for their support and patience.

*Special Thanks:* The inspiration that is Laird Henry. To O'Salvation I do pledge my fealty.

# PREFACE

We live in a Digital Babylon, in a world saturated by hard data and new technologies, insatiable for the pleasures of fresh images of our universe and of our selves. A milieu wherein the cinema has become, as Mike Figgis has pointed out, "the most oversubscribed whore in the art world."

Even so, wondering why one is drawn towards that flickering motion picture in the dark is akin to analyzing why one is drawn towards dreaming, or religion, or magic, or love. There are rationales and hard realities, but it is a passion beyond reason. It is that ineffable something that takes us beyond ourselves into another realm. And those who weave the tale, binding us with word, gesture and image, into that other world, vaunt an immense responsibility and a power.

A persuasive image can be perceived as truth, and therefore a reality, but even pre-cinematic visionaries as varied as Buddha, Scheherazade, the Marquis de Sade, Neitzsche and Shakespeare would all undoubtedly agree, that absolute truth itself is a concept with uncountable human variables.

This is not to say that we don't all love the Hollywood dog and pony show. Money. Power. Glossy, high-concept desire. Film trailers, pumping sex, promising satisfaction in under ninety minutes. Filmmakers idealized as all knowing gods. Performers flinging out their deepest cleavage on entertainment news programs for the sake of the weekend box office. Explosive genre films, mass-produced and cloned like hot buttered popcorn at a rate that would make Dolly the Sheep proud. Entertaining? You betcha.

Uplifting, inspiring? Well, then we curve back to the individuating precepts of reality and truth.

Which isn't to deny any of the hard work or joy or creative invention therein. There is also greatness to be found in trashy films, in those rock-'em-sock-'em blockbuster features. But if you were to hail their offspring as singular, well, that would be grasping—they don't call Hollywood the business capitol of entertainment for nothing. Its very girth, skill and reach has regularly and capably crushed those smaller, more unusual movies that might otherwise have found a way to sneak into your local multiplex.

But for a few exceptions, "off the rack" Hollywood film stories—and even much of what supposes to be fresh, independent cinema—have lulled us into mediocrity and acceptance. Much like fast food; once a low rent, lustful joy, now a familiar, comforting staple with half the required nutrients and vitamins. Bottom line: a movie may be loads of fun and do tremendous box office, but don't let that convince you it is the cinematic recreation of the Guttenberg Bible.

Celluloid is far from dead. But filmmakers who haven't been able to access the pricier tools of cinema, or those who wish to step off the main road for a while and explore, are now given a wider swathe in which to create, and an arena in which their work can be seen. And as more and more seasoned auteurs legitimize the medium, stepping behind the DV lens for a look-see, that formerly shabby second cousin to celluloid is looking like a one fabulous and sexy cinematic beast.

Yet, art and modern cinema are not mutually exclusive. And with the advent of DV filmmaking, and the provoking production concept of Dogme 95—a ten point vow of cinematic purity cooked up by Danish filmmakers Lars von Trier and Thomas Vinterberg—a new wave of images and experimental ideas have come to the fore, challenging the terrain of independent and Hollywood filmmaking on all levels. And quite possibly giving rise to a regeneration of pure form once again.

Yet—beyond commerce, beyond who has the biggest propheteer in town—for the people who love film, it is still all about that ineffable something. Storytellers wielding the camera, even in this gizmo-delirious Age of Technopia, stand as part of an age-old, mythological inheritance. They are the jesters, the magicians, the shaman shape shifters, the image tricksters, the disrupters of the status quo. Count Harmony Korine's irreverent foreword to this book, a very personal manifesto on the art of filmmaking which he calls his "comprehensive and forthright guide to mistakist cinema," in that long, provocative tradition.

As William Blake, said, "If the doors of perception were cleansed every thing would appear to man as it is, infinite." To have the capacity to explore the imagination's remote frontiers and the unmapped areas of the collective human unconsciousness is a gift. And every person within these pages, their individual fame and genius, their stance on art and film notwithstanding, reveals themselves to bound in that way, as by their deep, abiding passion for cinema. Their willingness to stumble in the process of that exploration is energizing and inspiring beyond measure.

And that's not just once upon a time.

[A comprehensive and forthright guide to "mistakist cinema"]

{The life and opinions}/Tristam shandy;

truth/lies- "the greatest novel of all time will be a novel that consists entirely of others quotations. Without any credit of origin unless, unless the credit is given purposefully to an incorrect author, ant-iauthorship/lie, used expressly for the purpose of confusing the reader. Or to get all the hippies off your front lawn."

~~Bonnie 'prince' billie- (if I could fuck a mountain, oh I would fuck a mountain, And I'd do it with women in the valley. If she comes Tumbling to me, seems every night there for me, with a different face and legs that will not quit.)~~

Scenario b-science project where the explosion is documented. Aktionists. Nitche et al muller,otto, commune nazi shittel collective.

(eustache killed himself after he made the mother and the whore 219 mn long.)

doctor- 1. gunner ficher hence sven nike.

(every man for himself and god against all_)

1. im feeling under the weather
2. so am i.
3. do you have a father?
4. yes.

Spielberg made the haulicaust in the image of E.T.

Deconstruction- joyce
Bishop to pope to ordetts - [carl theodore turn of the dreyer} the passion that never ceased)

Digi fuck digi cocaine, cameras, fuck all, slit wrists and francis bacon with a tattoo that sys brevity is the - of wit. It's a tool. Video is a tool that is all and your revolution can fuck itself.

Laird henn- whenever the truth is uncovered, the artist will always cling with rapt gaze to what still remains covering even after such uncovering; but the theoretical man enjoys and finds pleasure in the discarded covering and finds the highest object of his pleasure in the process of an ever happening uncovering that succeeds through his own efforts.

A prelude-wagner or Finnegan's wake.

cocaine is not a vitamin for the prophetic experimentalists of the day. My walter Benjamin had jaundice cheeks but wrote the arcades project with hitler on his shoulders.

Camcorder the corner on the grace kelly, light camera, forgot what to say. All the filmmakers but some, say their prayers.

> The dogme 95.
> (I thought brothers share blood.)
> Do my Dane brethren care if I was to die tomorrow?
> I must confess. Do I?

4c- RELAPSE- this art, cinema, if it is, I know it can and has been, has stolen and destroyed far more then it has fulfilled me. It has helped to reinforce my disdain for the simple-minded viewer. The brainwashed slug who believes in nothing. The director must have faith in god because he who truly understands the power makes the life abound.

The future is here and it is shit, and it is smiles on the posters, and worst of all the enemy of the future is emotion. To feel is to die. And most sitting in the dark are dead. And happy to be dead. I understand nothing about what the people want, nothing. *i wish i could.*

Detox - I want no answers. Only your mistakes can save me.

*deism-* Creation 101 years /or how edison destroyed god – when the camera projected at 24 frames, man looked and saw himself on the screen. He saw himself in big. It wasn't until the cinema that man actually saw who he thought he was and or who he wanted to be. And until that point in time man had thought of god in mainly simple, comfortable terms, we had to visualize him. God to us was big and he had no compitition. Now that we are the same size as god, we don't need him, he is worthless to us, we can sit in the movie house/temple on Sundays. God will commit your suicide. The virgin mary is bardot. God has left us here with 32 elvis movies all dubbed in german.

*Bresson-* ~~Kill yourself when your tired~~, sniffed heroin off the top of a golf cart in the summer of 69 the year I one the pulitzer.

I am one of gods ~~spent~~ "mistakes."

Laird henn
(formerly harmony korine)

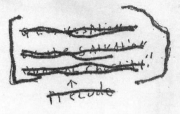

IDIOTS
VS.
~~Boy~~ V.S. Celebration
JULIEN DONKEY 329

LArs        So

I'll shout: I WUV OO!
[TO COMMITTEE]        Don't you bastards smile!

LAIRD

Again.

I WUV OO YEWWY MUCH!
[TO BROTHER-IN-LAW]        And I'll

LArs

break your grinning head if you don't get
it out of here!

Oo mean I'm free?

LArs                        I'll bet
I tear you limb from limb, you funking boozer!

~~VINTEBERG~~        Hah. You always were a lousy lover.        [Exits

CRITIC        So what do we do now, ~~_____~~?
LAIRD

Don't ask me. I should've stayed in bed
this morning.

That's my boy! Come on, let's rush.

LArS        What about ~~_____~~ SPIELBERG?
LAIRD        to be accused of parricide—and worse!

Forget that old hermaphrodite. The curse
of every campus is its local prophet.
Tell him he should take his charge and stuff it.

VINTEBERG        Mercy, how unorthodox a view!

All right, so it's unorthodox. So sue
LAIRD        me, Look, I'll prove to you once and for all
what Ibars proph-proj's are: one came to call
on us and my first husband years ago,
LArS        just after we were married, and you know
what he told ~~_____~~ would be his fortune.

LUCAS

Laird        What?

He said I'd better get an abortion
quick, or else my husband would be killed
LArs        by his own son.

And was that curse fulfilled?

LAIRD        Of course not, silly! Naturally I declared
the proph-proj was a liar; but he scared
~~_____~~ so bad that when our kid
Lars        was born—a boy—we secretly got rid
of him the way unmarried co-eds do it.

And how was that, I wonder?

Laird                        Nothing to it:
we stuck a peg or something in his feet
and dumped him in the woods for crows to eat.

[page 95 discussion]

Q– What is the future of DV.
cinema?

A– DV
mixed
with
cocaine
injections
~~And ChiNese~~
~~abortions~~

its about what you bring to the table Not eat at the table
for the first time a person can improvise
alone in camera in much the same way
so called free Jazz came to be. A Natural Progression
With an audience who doesnt care to see any true
cinematic progression. Film as Art is an idea whose
time has come to pass. Could a master Like Bergman even
Be able to get his films Financed today? Never

3

### The mistakist manifest

This is obviously for those of us who have made a dogme film or one day will. Although I had nothing to do with the vow of chastity autorship I would like to propose a less cosmetic attempt.

1. no plots. Only images. Stories are fine
2. all edits affects in camera only.
3. 600 cameras/ A WALL OF Pictures / the Phil Spector of cine'

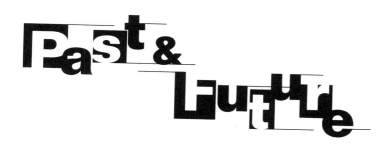

# Past & Future

*Jean-Luc Godard* **france**
THE FUTURE OF CINEMA

*I am something of a loner. I am partnered with my friend Anne-Marie Miéville in a small production company, and have little contact with young filmmakers. Never had any. I've always considered myself marginal. I see fewer films. I no longer live in Paris. The city has grown too big, with too many grays, too much dust, too many gas fumes. I try to follow the release of films but when you don't live in Paris.... Only in Paris, and thanks to the influence of the New Wave, can one see films from everywhere in the world, even if they're only shown for a week in a minuscule theater. However, on the rare occasion when I have met some of them, with one or two exceptions, I had the feeling I was younger—or dumber—than they were. Not as a man, but as a filmmaker.*

*I've always been interested in technique, not in art for technique's sake. In the last installments of* History of Cinema, *I keep saying—or often have it said—that cinema is neither an art nor a technique, but a mystery. That's what dif-*

# The cinema is not an ART which films LIFE: the cinema is something *B*ETWEEN art and life.

ferentiates it from painting, literature or music; all arts when undertaken by artists. Cinema is close to a religion. It is somewhat an act of faith. It is immediately perceivable, through photography, or a certain relationship between man and the world—is the world the work of man or vice-versa? I don't know. The two go together.... One could say television has "un-taught" us to see. Television manufactures a few memories, but cinema—as it should have been—creates memory, i.e. the possibility of memory.

Video has its own specificity. It can be used for its uniqueness, but, in my opinion, rarely is. On video, I love doing superimpositions, real superimpositions, almost as in music, where movements mix—sometimes slowly, sometimes brutally—then something happens. You can have two images at the same time, much like you can have two ideas at the same time, and you can commute between the two, which, to me, seems very close to childhood. One of its main interests is that you can work at it at home, if you can afford it or have a production company that allows you to do so. You can therefore work a bit more, perhaps, like a painter or a musician, and realize that the image is not only space but also time.

Although, hopefully, I still have a fair number of years to live, I hope the police won't force me to use a computer. Don't forget that highways were invented by Adolf Hitler and a few others of the same ilk. I don't think a highway helps knowing

and appreciating a landscape. Same thing, for me, applies to the "information highway." In today's configuration of cinema, I think my films and those of Jean-Marie Straub, Jean Vigo and John Cassavetes may be less seen than they used to be, since it's technology—CD-ROMs, the Internet—that will determine "the classics," the "necessary" films, unless cinemathèques and film archives manage to protect them, but they're so weak, and cinema is not, like painting, a "fine" art. No cinemathèque can be as successful as the Louvre Museum, simply because cinema, as it was born, and born only 100 years ago, is still a mechanical art.

## Unlike painting and literature, the cinema both G I V *E* S to life and T *A* K E S from it, and I try to render this concept in my films.

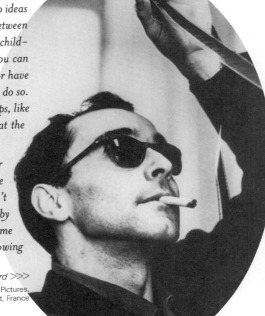

*Jean-Luc Godard* >>>
courtesy of Rialto Pictures,
New York City; Gaumont, France

Very early on, however, audiences gave an extraordinarily warm welcome to cinema, the likes of which they never bestowed on any other form of art. But what was immediately privileged was the "spectacular," the "commercial" aspect of it—in the worst sense of the word, for "commerce" is also a necessary component of it all. For me, cinema is a metaphor for the world. It is image, and as such, it was an image of something. Everything is image, in the largest sense of the word.

There was a time when you distributed what you produced. Distribution was at the service of production. You produced and then distributed what you had produced. Nowadays, you produce in order to distribute. When France celebrates "the 100th Anniversary of cinema," what is actually being celebrated is the 100th anniversary of the first performance in front of a paying audience. I think it is wonderful to pay $3, $10, $20 to see something on a wide screen. Then make it clear that that's the marvel you're celebrating. Whereas there is another wonder, and that is the work itself. But maybe people have a lesser need of wonderment

in their lives; maybe wars on television are enough for them.

Cinema is what it will become, what the public or the filmgoers as a whole will want it to be. It could be something else but, you know, man, nature, the nature of man...You can't spend your life saying, "It was better in my younger days." But at the beginning, cinema was a tool for study. It should have been a tool for study—for it is visual, and very close to science and medicine. The camera has a lens, like a microscope, to study the infinitely small, or like a telescope, to study the infinitely distant. Having studied that, you could then convey it in a spectacular fashion.

The work of a filmmaker is to try and make his film as best he can. Contrary to what is often said, a camera is not a gun, and a gun is not a camera: if it were, they wouldn't still blindfold those who are about to be shot.

(Godard's newest work, Éloge de l'Amour, premiered at the 2001 Cannes Film Festival)

The truth is that there is no terror untempered by some great moral idea.
OUTSIDE of content, and content the INSIDE of style. To me style is just the outside and the inside of the HUMAN body. Both go together, they can't be separated.

# NEW OLD WAVES D INFLUENCES

As with all the arts, filmmaking is a deeply biased process of image and ideological selection that has evolved gradually over the years. Films and filmmakers will always quote, compare, borrow from and surpass each other, and in doing so, continually reinvent and reevaluate cinema's history.

Below is my own highly partisan list of twenty directors and their comedies, musicals, melodramas and documentaries which have influenced today's filmmakers.

## 1. THE NIGHT OF THE HUNTER (1955)

Director: Charles Laughton. Before *Blair Witch*, there was Robert Mitchum's fanatical preacher with LOVE/HATE tattooed on his knuckles. Psychological unrest doesn't come close to describing the emotional punch of Laughton's only directorial effort, and nothing touches the unforgettable shot of the dead Shelley Winters floating at the bottom of the river like a waterlogged Ophelia, her hair drifting as aimlessly as seaweed.

## 2. PUTNEY SWOPE (1969)

Director: Robert Downey. A precursor to Spike Lee's satire *Bamboozled*, and considered *trés* avant-garde at the time, Downey Sr.'s ultracool spoof of blaxploitation and black power has a very punk rock ethos even though it occurred almost a decade before the Ramones or the Sex Pistols. This was a movie that proved you could do nearly anything in cinema, and it didn't necessarily have to make sense. Outrageous, politically abrasive and frequently hilarious, this film spoke to the counterculture's hopes for what underground film could accomplish. Its political edge remains sharp and cutting.

## 3. MAN WITH A MOVIE CAMERA (1929)

Director: Dziga Vertov. Early cinematic improvisation found its hero in this Soviet revolutionary filmmaker. The constructivist prankster used to make his film crew practice shooting with no film in the camera! When he actually used stock, Vertov was able to capture some remarkably fresh images. Out and about on the streets of Moscow, circa 1929, Vertov documents a day in the life of the city and its people; children laughing, cityscapes, weddings, childbirth, factories at work and motorcycle riders racing down the track. This dialogue-free film blurs into a collage of images, linking the mechanical to the organic. One can't help but see traces of Vertov in Harmony Korine's *julien donkey-boy*, wherein Korine and DP Anthony Dod Mantle wield their intimate array of DV spy cameras, stealing their way into shops, buses and behind closed doors.

## 4. NASHVILLE (1975)

Director: Robert Altman. The first great ensemble picture—and huge influence on Paul Thomas Anderson's *Magnolia*, and certainly Jennifer Jason Leigh and Alan Cumming's *The Anniversary Party*—*Nashville* is a consummate Cinemascope movie; incredibly bold with its extended camera takes, overlapping dialogue and the multi-track recording that Altman first implemented here. The director juggles multiple stories without antagonizing the audience. The film feels natural, dirty and messy, but remains very cutting-edge. One of Altman's best—right up there with *The Long Goodbye*.

## 5. PULL MY DAISY (1959)

Directors: Robert Frank/Alfred Leslie. Ethan Hawke's Dylan Thomas-inspired *Chelsea Walls* certainly took a slice of 'tude from this flick. Only a half-hour long, this Beat classic is one of the most casually hip flicks in the world. Featuring a voiceover by Jack Kerouac, and appearances by Beat poetry icons Allen Ginsberg and Gregory Corso, you can practically smell the weed and narcissism lurking under the principals' cooler-than-thou exteriors.

## 6. TOUCH OF EVIL (1958)

Director: Orson Welles. The fat man returneth. Welles, well past his *Citizen Kane* prime and waistline, chews the scenery as a corrupt Mexican policeman, making life miserable for border cop Charlton Heston and his virginal new gringa bride, Janet Leigh. Marlene Dietrich has all the best lines as a raven-haired fortuneteller. Keep this film in mind when you watch Nic Cage trying to make his way out of town in John Dahl's *Red Rock West*.

## 7. GOODFELLAS (1990)

Director: Martin Scorsese. He is one of Allison Anders' idols and it's not hard to guess why. Performance-wise, *Goodfellas* is amazing, but it also borrows techniques from French filmmakers

**"Digitizing actors?** I find it highly unlikely. If you create actors, then you get into an area of inventing performance. There could be advantages, of course. We wouldn't have to get up as early. You could end up doing more than one movie at a time. You wouldn't have to turn down a movie because you were already working—you could just create another of you digitally—a better version, of course. From a filmmaking point of view, I think most filmmakers would applaud, knowing you could create actors.... But then you get into an area of inventing performance. I don't know if we'll get that far...in terms of the digital world, probably the aspect that most filmmakers are going to encourage is digital projection because there isn't a filmmaker around hasn't seen reel four of his or her film go green or yellow. That's very often the most frustrating thing about doing a movie, and making a studio film. The first 100 prints may be of quality, but the rest of them are pretty bad. I think for quality, the sheer desire of the filmmaker to want the tone, the color of the film image of a film to be as exact as you want, digital is the way to go."

KEVIN SPACEY / director, *Albino Alligator*; producer, *The Big Kahuna*; actor, *American Beauty* like Truffaut, interpreted by a director at the peak of his craft. Bravura all the way through. The long traveling shot into the Copacabana you can trace back to Max Ophuls. Obnoxious and brilliant in equal measure are the pretentious, insane camera moves that suddenly all make perfect sense.

### 8. THE FOREIGNER (1978)

Director: Amos Poe. Before Gus Van Sant hit his stride with *Drugstore Cowboy* (1989), he was soaking in the loopy, gritty reality of the low-budget indie kings, the Kuchar Brothers, Andy Warhol and Poe. Straight from New York, made in the era of the Ramones and Talking Heads, *The Foreigner* is one of the first of its genre. Made for about $5,000 and featuring Debbie Harry as gorgeous hooker, it is loose and raw, close to the spirit of late '70s punk music where musicianship wasn't important, and virtuosity was not the main criterion, it was simply, "I have something I want to express." A highly original punk rock movie.

### 9. CONTEMPT (1963)

Director: Jean Luc Godard. Cited by all as a major influence (even Quentin Tarantino, who dubbed his production company A Band Apart after the director's 1964 film *Bande á part*). Subverting the typical narrative by using all the handsome old tools, Godard's early films—*Breathless, My Life to Live, A Married Woman, Masculine-Feminine*—were acerbic love stories set in Parisian cafes, of men and women talking, arguing, smoking and polemicizing their lives away. This is hardly Godard's riskiest work. Although it does feature Brigitte Bardot at her most glorious, it exposes Godard's feelings for the seductive lie of movies. A canny guerrilla to the end, Godard never lets you forget film is a very expensive art, and cinema is his way to continue his cultural assaults on the status quo.

### 10. SINGIN' IN THE RAIN (1952)

Director: Stanley Donen. There's Ernst Lubitsch's *The Merry Widow* (1934) of course, but it is the glory of *Singin' in the Rain* which partially inspired Lars von Trier's "musical," *Dancer in the Dark* (the other film is Richard Brooks' *In Cold Blood* [1967]). It's full of everything you want to see when you go to see a movie musical—beautiful people, bimbos, cigar-chomping studio execs...and it's colorful and funny to boot. And not only does it have a great story about the transition from silent film to talkies, Gene Kelly's "Singin' in the Rain" number and Donald O'Connor, when he dances in "Make 'em Laugh," are flat-out amazing.

## 11. SHOOT THE PIANO PLAYER (1960)

Director: Francois Truffaut. *The 400 Blows* aside, here you have Truffaut's penultimate gangster movie. He took the old American tough-guy movie, all that Humphrey Bogart ethos, and turned it on its ear. The people in this film aren't classically handsome, but they are sexy and cool. It was shot in Cinemascope, usually reserved for big budget Hollywood movies. Reinventing the genre, and taking it somewhere brand-new and post-modern; our hero could be a little skinnier and not so tough. One of the funniest, most notorious moments is when one of the characters says, "May my grandmother drop dead if I'm telling a lie right now," and it cuts immediately to a shot of his grandmother dropping to the floor, dead. Then it immediately cuts back as if nothing had happened. Clearly a touch-stone for filmmakers as wide-ranging as *Being John Malkovich* scribe Charlie Kaufman to the Farrelly Brothers (*There's Something About Mary*).

## 12. FACES (1968)

Director: John Cassavetes. There are many wonderful films by Cassavetes (*Shadows* [1961], *A Woman Under the Influence* [1974]), but this is the one where you really feel his heart. Perhaps it has to do with the sublime acting and ravishing beauty of his star, muse and wife, Gena Rowlands. Worshipped and emulated by 2K directors around the globe for his entire oeuvre, *Faces* is improvisational Cassavetes at his finest. A look at the dissolution of a middle-class, married couple's fourteen-year marriage over a day and a half, *Faces* lingers on emotional issues with a nervy documentary fervor.

## 13. MELVIN AND HOWARD (1980)

Director: Jonathan Demme. Demme is *Chuck & Buck* director Miguel Arteta's idol. His films have rough edges, perfectly crafted. Some elements seem slightly off in certain moments, but are perfectly modulated and meant to be there. Consider the first twenty minutes: Two guys talking in a car. That's it. It's stunning the way the movie sets you up to accept whatever happens. This one hits the emotional bullseye, especially when it comes to Paul Le Mat's amazing turn as a sweetheart of a loser who just misses a break.

## 14. THEY LIVE BY NIGHT (1948)

Director: Nicholas Ray. Avoiding man-on-the-run clichés, and carrying considerable emotional impact instead, it's based on Edward Anderson's *Thieves Like Us* (remade by Robert Altman in 1974 under the same name). Capturing emotional malaise through his poetic use of space, not only is this Ray's first film, it's still one of the most romantic and haunting young-lovers-on-the-run movies ever made. Jim Jarmusch, who calls Ray one of his heroes, once worked as his teaching assistant at NYU Film School.

## 15. STRAY DOG (1949)

Director: Akira Kurosawa. George Lucas thinks the world of this legendary auteur, and it's easy to see why. Hollywood may have co-opted Kurosawa's mythic storytelling style, but few can emulate his genius. This film has a plot you can describe in one sentence: a rookie cop loses his gun and has to get

**"As an actor,** you do a scene one time, and then you know they're going to set up to shoot it on this side of the room and you know you have until after lunch to think about what you're really going to do with the scene. [With a DV movie] the level of preparation—it's so rapid fire, you need to be much more prepared. There won't be that afternoon. ❖ It's very easy to attract actors, it's always very simple. No matter what level of film you're working on, [the way to do it] is with good writing. Acting is an interpretative art and your performance is only as good as the writing. If you're working on Chekhov, it's your job to match him. If you're working on some silly TV show, it's your job to raise it up, and I think in general, digital films allow for a higher level of experimentation in the writing, which actors find attractive. What DV has [also] done is make it almost as cheap to make a movie as it is to write a book, or to paint. There is the possibility that there will be a glut, that they'll be lots of garbage.... I compare it with something like Kerouac's *On the Road*, which you read as a teen and it makes you think, "I can write a book!" Or like Cassavetes' *Shadows*—"I can make a movie!" There's something really beautiful about that. I shot my movie and it looks like a DV picture, that is the aesthetic. I wanted to accent what it was capable of. Some people shoot theirs to look like film. It works the way works. Is Jackson Pollock the same as Van Gogh? No; it's all different. The question is, is the project succeeding? Does it tell a story? Is it becoming a piece of art? I really feel it is an especially exciting time to be alive, to be working. The possibilities are endless."
ETHAN HAWKE / actor,
*Tape*; director,
*Chelsea Walls*

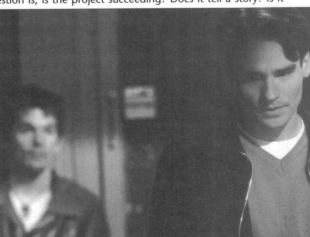

>>>
*Ethan Hawke (l) and Robert Sean Leonard (r) in* Tape.
courtesy of Lions Gate Films

it back. That's it. He sets out to recover the weapon by going under-cover for a while in the city's "lower depths." This movie opens, immediately, literally, with a bang. The first shot is a close-up of a guy saying, "I lost my gun." The funny thing is, while Truffaut in France was ripping off American gangster movies, Kurosawa in Japan was doing the same thing nearly a decade before. They're both loving Howard Hawks, Raoul Walsh and John Ford, then taking them back home, mixing it up, and taking it to another level.

## 16. BRANDED TO KILL (1967)

Director: Seijun Suzuki. Tongue-in-cheek shoot-em-up Director Robert Rodriquez (*El Mariachi, Desperado, Spy Kids*) must've picked up a few tips from this man. A generation after Kurosawa, Suzuki gives us this surrealist, witty film. Replete with gouge-your-eyes-out gorgeous composition, this is the ultimate '60s Japanese hit-man movie; both incomprehensible and exhilarat-ing. The plot, about an assassin-for-hire who has been targeted for elimination, is impossible to understand on the first viewing and irrelevant on subsequent ones. The film's setpieces, howev-er, are mesmerizing. The gunman launches a balloon and times its ascent so he can kill somebody in a high-rise, jump out the window to escape, and accomplish both without hurting himself.

## 17. BAD DAY AT BLACK ROCK (1955)

Director: John Sturges. This film is very simple in its storytelling. Spencer Tracy's perform-ance is the quintessential. The phrase that is always used to describe him is: "He's not doing anything and it's perfect." The other great thing about this film is its dialogue. It balances what is real, and what it really sounds like, with the way we talk and communicate. Alexander McKendrick's *Sweet Smell of Success* (1957) a few years later had the same amazing syntax and rhythm. Neil LaBute (*In the Company of Men, Your Friends and Neighbors, Nurse Betty*), who knows a thing or two about the dark side of human emotion, has nothing on this baby. Playwright Clifford Odets (*Golden Boy*) wrote the script and it is one the most cynical movies ever written.

### 18. DON'T LOOK BACK (1967)

Director: D.A. Pennebaker. Wim Wenders' *Buena Vista Social Club* brought Cuban rhythms and DV lit to the mainstream, but three decades before, we worshipped at the throne of the young and snotty Dylan, in rough, beautifully grainy black-and-white. One of the best rock 'n' roll movies ever made and the model for all rock poseurs to follow. Featuring a luminous Joan Baez, *Don't Look Back* reveals that Dylan, alas, has feet of clay like all the rest of us. He is immature, petty, vindictive and lacking a sense of humor. You can't take your eyes off him.

### 19. THE GODFATHER (1972)

Director: Francis Ford Coppola. A juicy cinematic offer that can't be refused, this epic tale of a family soiled by secrets and lies put the Corleone clan on the map, and Coppola in the catbird seat. Marlon Brando was in a slump when he was hired for this picture, but his mumbling, marbles-in-the-mouth performance launched a thousand parodies and earned him an Oscar®. Later that same year he got even chancier with Bernardo Bertolucci's *Last Tango in Paris* (1972). Still considered to be a landmark feature, *The Godfather* is also one of the films that *The Celebration* director Thomas Vinterberg cites as inspiration (the other is Ingmar Bergman's *Fanny and Alexander* [1983]).

### 20. BLOW UP (1966)

Director: Michelangelo Antonioni. Influential to all budding auteurs, the eye of the camera comes center stage in this classic '60s art film. Starring David Hemmings as a hip London fashion photographer who unwittingly photographs a murder that may involve a young and gorgeous Vanessa Redgrave, *Blow Up* forces the viewer to share the protagonist's confusion as to what he saw, or thinks he saw. The wandering plot takes viewers through a "swinging" London, rife with hashish, sex, nubile fashion models (including Jean Shrimpton) and concludes with an imaginary volleyball game played by mimes. A mystery movie where the mystery actually grows more mysterious, and then simply ceases. Even Mike Meyers took a stroll through Antonioni's wiggy *mise en scene* with his *Austin Powers: International Man of Mystery* (1997).

> "The Steve Spielberg of today is not using 8mm, he's using High 8 digital and he doesn't have to beg his father for another roll of film because he can usually take it out of his lunch money."
>
> **GEORGE LUCAS** / writer/director/producer, *Star Wars* trilogy

**ALSO RECOMMENDED:**

1. *The Passion of Saint Joan* (1928) Carl Dreyer
2. *Peeping Tom* (1960) Michael Powell
3. *Raging Bull* (1980) Martin Scorsese
4. *Love Streams* (1984) John Cassavetes
5. *Dead Ringers* (1988) David Cronenberg
6. *Women in Love* (1970) Ken Russell
7. *The Road Warrior* (1982) George Miller
8. *Toute une Nuit* (1982) Chantal Akerman
9. *Do the Right Thing* (1989) Spike Lee
10. *The Flavor of Green Tea over Rice* (1952) Yasujiro Ozu
11. *A Clockwork Orange* (1971) Stanley Kubrick
12. *Sherlock, Jr.* (1924) Buster Keaton
13. *Bob le Flambeur* (1955) Jean-Pierre Melville
14. *Performance* (1970) Nicolas Roeg & Donald Cammell
15. *Point Blank* (1967) John Boorman
16. *A Hard Day's Night* (1964) Richard Lester
17. *The Story of the Last Chrysanthemums* (1939) Kenji Mizoguchi
18. *Straw Dogs* (1972) Sam Peckinpah
19. *Village of the Damned* (1960) Wolf Rilla
20. *The Big Heat* (1953) Fritz Lang
21. *Pickpocket* (1959) Robert Bresson
22. *Distant Voices, Still Lives* (1988) Terence Davies
23. *Faster Pussycat! Kill! Kill!* (1966) Russ Meyer
24. *Un Chant d'Amour* (1950) Jean Genet
25. *Life Is Sweet* (1990) Mike Leigh
26. *Nosferatu* (1922) F.W. Murnau
27. *Medium Cool* (1969) Haskell Wexler
28. *E.T. The Extra Terrestrial* (1982) Steven Spielberg
29. *Annie Hall* (1977) Woody Allen
30. *High Noon* (1952) Fred Zinnemann
31. *City Lights* (1931) Charlie Chaplin
32. *The Red Shoes* (1948) Michael Powell, Emeric Pressburger
33. *Sunrise* (1927) F.W. Murnau
34. *Brazil* (1985) Terry Gilliam
35. *Withnail and I* (1987) Bruce Robinson
36. *The Company of Wolves* (1984) Neil Jordan
37. *San Soliel* (1982) Chris Marker
38. *Un Chien Andalou* (1929) Luis Buñuel
39. *A Death in Venice* (1971) Luchino Visconti
40. *Metropolis* (1926) Fritz Lang

41. *One from the Heart* (1982) Francis Ford Coppola

42. *Sid and Nancy* (1986) Alex Cox

43. *Orpheus* (1949) Jean Cocteau

44. *Fail Safe* (1964) Sidney Lumet

45. *The Texas Chainsaw Massacre* (1975) Tobe Hooper

46. *Heart of Glass* (1976) Werner Herzog

47. *The Marriage of Maria Braun* (1979) Rainer Werner Fassbinder

48. *Hiroshima, Mon Amour* (1959) Alain Resnais

49. *Celine and Julie Go Boating* (1974) Jacques Rivette

50. *Rules of the Game* (1939) Jean Renoir

# HOLLYWOOD

# INDIEWOOD AND REALITY

Squint around. Voyeurism and capitalism are everywhere the imagination can reach. Video cameras positioned in private homes stream "real-time" lives to your laptop; high quality pro-sumer cameras transform dewy-eyed cineastes with computer editing software into 2K auteurs; DV "reality" images compete with popular TV and film devices; Hollywood plotters churn out ultra-cheap shot-on-video cinema in the name of art, as well as cutting out the middlemen via Internet downloading of films to sites as far afield as Malaysia. The nature of reality is no longer existential mumbo jumbo, it's the jingle in your pocket and the dream of stardom in your heart.

George Lucas, who swoons at the crystalline perfection of the 24P high-definition camera (as does his *Star Wars - Episode I: The Phantom Menace* [2000]), proclaimed that all-digital movie pro-duction would make filmmaking more democratic. Clearly, the big boys didn't always feel this way, although Francis Ford Coppola has been fascinated by "electronic cinema" ever since DP Vittorio Storraro lensed his amazing (albeit financially dis-astrous) *One From the Heart* in 1982. The first mainstreamed phase of features shot utilizing video cameras were self-referencing whacks at the ancient tree of cinematic beauty. Cheapening the brilliance of celluloid with their tarty lighting, *Candid Camera* associations and adolescent camerawork, they always needed to find a way to involve the camera itself. In its higher state, the zeitgeist informed Steven Soderbergh's *sex, lies and videotape* (1989). In its lower state it was appropriated by slasher movies and ribald teen excursions, as if subtextually apologizing for its shameful intrusion and rubbishy likenesses of authenticity.

The root of these pseudo-vérité truths, lensed as wobbly, stranger-than-fiction narratives, had a prescient punch which eventually served up the homegrown success of *The Blair Witch Project* (1999), which cost $40,000 to make and grossed over $140 million. At the other end of the spectrum, gracefully transmogrified by DP Conrad Hall's Oscar®-winning 35mm lens, is *American Beauty* (1999), modestly budgeted at $15 million. Most importantly in the eyes of the industry: both made money.

Meanwhile, before we were counting up the boxoffice receipts, halfway across the world, in Europe—which spangle-eyed Americans perceive as the paradigm of serious filmmaking—there was an ideology brewing via a Danish born, DV led aesthetic; Dogme 95. Created under a monastic, ten-point rule system the Calvinists might have partied around, it launched Dogme #1, *The Celebration* (1998), in which the disintegrated imagery of a one-chip DV camera brutally underscored the disintegration of a damaged family; and Dogme #2, *The Idiots* (1998), shot on a three-chip Sony VX1000, a heavily improvised, Bergmanesque excursion about a collective of overly privileged postmodern hippies who pose as idiots to unburden themselves of the crushing restraints of a politically correct society. The former struck a chord, won an award at Cannes, and was hailed for bravura storytelling. Less of a crowd pleaser, the latter was a mordant victory for its famously rigid auteur. Neither one contained a subplot about a film being made to validate its handheld video aesthetic.

> "*Traffic* is my $49 million handheld Dogme film."
> **STEVEN SODERBERGH** / director, *Traffic, Erin Brockovich, Ocean's 11*

Widely perceived as either a high-concept joke or a return to creative purity, and possibly both, Dogme 95 has always received mixed reviews. For the teeming DV masses, it legitimized the digital aesthetic as a viable new wave and tipped scores of indie idealists to the possibility of a grassroots filmmaking that played with the medium, if not necessarily by the rules. DV projects from established filmmakers such as Wim Wenders (*Buena Vista Social Club*, 1998) and Mike Figgis (*TimeCode*, 2000) only added to its freshly-minted sex appeal.

**"Technology** is always out there as a danger for upstaging the story. I mean, technology was out there as a danger even in the old days when they had to pull mattes the old fashioned way. So the same rules apply. This simply makes your imagination easier to capture and present. And when you think about it, more economical to present an impossible idea. Ten years ago, nobody would pay for the impossible to go up on the screen, today, with this technology you can pretty much explore the depths of your imagination and express yourself any way you like. With everyone going digital throughout the world, it's important that kids don't come into the real world without the tools and knowledge of how to apply their talent inside a world that's rapidly changing technologically."

**STEVEN SPIELBERG** / writer/director/producer, *A.I.*; director/producer, *Jaws, Raiders of the Lost Ark*

Historically, low budget filmmaking has been the only way for many neophytes to launch themselves into Hollywood careers from humble beginnings at the 7-11. During the 1970s and 1980s, there were micro-budgeted features such as Jim Jarmusch's *Stranger Than Paradise* and Spike Lee's *She's Gotta Have It*. And following similar byways, in the 1990s debut films such as Rick Linklater's *Slacker*, Robert Rodriguez's *El Mariachi*, Kevin Smith's *Clerks* and Neil LaBute's *In the Company of Men* established a new modus vivendi for other filmmakers.

Co-opting the ethos on a grander scale, Hollywood is tapping into the nerve of the ever-burgeoning digital revolution at breakneck speed. Despite its superior beauty, the charms of celluloid are pricey. The bottom line is that DV is cheaper, lasts longer, and eventually, when there are no more prints to be shipped, films can be beamed to the theaters from a Big Brother-like central terminal to multiplexes around the country. And that digi pie in the sky is coming up fast. Digital projecting systems are already in place at selected theaters, quietly introduced into film festivals, and screening video captured stories for audiences who never suspect the truth. Within five years (according to some triumphant anti-celluloid Luddites), those images etched into strips of film will be the stuff of dreamy nostalgia. But perhaps not. For now at least, we can continue to choose the way in which we dream in the dark.

# PRODUCERS COMMENTARY

## JASON KLIOT
### Open City Films and Blow Up Pictures

Blow Up Pictures, the digital production arm of Open City Films, headed by Jason Kliot and Joana Vicente, has been at the vanguard of the digital film-making movement since 1999. While Open City has recently produced such celluloid titles as Tony Bui's *Three Seasons*, Miramax's teen flick *Down to You*, and the upcoming *Love the Hard Way*, Blow Up's resume includes such intriguing films as Miguel Arteta's *Chuck & Buck* and Daniel Minahan's *Series 7*.

The team—which got its start as associate producers on *Welcome to the Dollhouse*—has bridged the gap between Indiewood and digi-indies in just a few years. In January 2001, the Lipsky Brothers' Lot 47 Films signed a distribution deal with Blow Up to release half of their features over the next three years. In return, they promised to give the Lipskys 50 percent of their new digital films with budgets of $1 million or less. Covering North American rights in all media, Blow Up hopes to explode into a "digital studio."

"A few years ago," says Kliot, "we were completely at the mercy of the mini-majors to get our product out there. With our Lot 47 deal, every single digital feature that we produce will be distributed theatrically in every major city in the U.S. with a very serious print and advertising commitment behind it." And that ain't just whistling indie.

**You already had Open City Films. Why did you create Blow Up Pictures?**

Our reason for starting Blow Up Pictures came out of a strong belief that American independent film was waning. We felt there was a real problem; that the studios had slowly been encroaching onto territory that independents had usually dominated. I'm speaking of the Hollywood version of an art movie...meaning *American Beauty*, *Being John Malkovich*.

**The way that big budget movies take the qualities of independent cinema and make them mass-market friendly?**

Yes. I really felt that meant the end of independent film. My partner Joana and I were also bemoaning the quality of scripts coming into our company, Open City. Most were written to get an actor attached, to get the writers into Sundance or to launch their careers in Hollywood. At the same time, as independent producers, we were giving away our souls in terms of final cuts for directors, creative control and all the things that make independent film truly unique. To us, producing means creating a space in which great art can be made. We were confident that there must be people out there who just wanted to make movies, who had to express themselves as artists.

We realized that in a way it was *The Celebration* that kindled it all…that it was possible to go out and shoot a digital feature for under $1 million that could look great and be well received. So we founded Blow Up Pictures in 1999. It was also the same year that *Three Seasons* won three awards at Sundance. It brought a lot of attention to us as the first company to really say, "We make digital features and we are listing the movies we are going to make this year," and then actually do it. We made three movies our first year—how many times does that happen? We made artistic films by talented people, focused entirely on content. *Chuck & Buck* and *Series 7* were screenplays that almost every producer in the country had seen. They were floating around for three or four years, but nobody had the guts to make these movies. How did we end up focusing on content? Because of our basic tenet: The director has final cut.

**That shows an awful lot of faith.**

We have no cast attachments required, either. The most corrupting problem in independent film is the casting. The second you start thinking, "Who should be in my movie so I can get it made?" you're thinking ass-backwards, instead of asking, "Is the script good?"

**What is your budget range?**

Right now we're not thinking above two million. *Chuck & Buck* was well under $1 million.

**Is this financially feasible? Don't you need a famous actress nude in your picture to guarantee foreign distribution?**

It's absolutely moronic thinking, but that recouping you are talking about does not happen a lot. Because if a movie doesn't have U.S. theatrical distribution and it isn't a genre movie.... Look, if you're making a movie that has a very simple theme to it, that an international buyer can understand, and you say, "Isabelle Adjani is in my film and she's flashing her boobs," then you can sell your movie. A well-known actor can help, if you have made a good movie, because he or she can promote your movie, but it has to be the *right* movie. But if Arnold Schwarznegger made an independent movie—not such a sure thing. Arnold means something if he makes *Terminator 5*. If Arnold makes an art film with a genre element it can hold, but if it's just art, it doesn't hold.

## What does it take for Blow Up to greenlight a picture?

We'll greenlight your movie, you can cast anybody in the world. If that person happens to be the director's best friend, we tell him what we think, but we let him do it. If you slip into "maybe my character doesn't have to be fifty, he can be thirty," and mindsets like that, you end up with a mediocre movie which has nothing to do with the vision of the person who originated it. But sometimes you have to play the casting game if you go beyond a certain budget, which is why we decided to split our company. Open City makes movies that are $3 million to $5 million and up; we're developing Miguel Arteta's next film with USA Films, Tony Bui's next, Mira Nair's next....

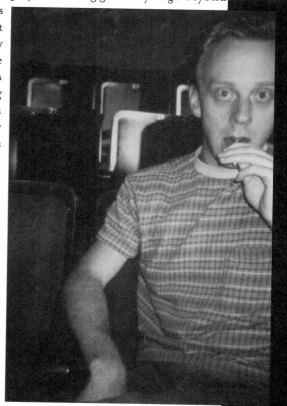

## Does the budget lead the aesthetic of these films?

Right now it does. With the 24P HD camera, that all could change. These cameras are more expensive, but people are willing to give us deals to get it done and a lot of companies want us to use their stuff, they want to be seen in our credits. So we do get breaks.

*Michael White as Buck in* Chuck & Buck.
courtesy of Blow Up Pictures/Artisan Entertainment,
photo by Alexia C. Pilat

**So you would lean towards 24P HD?**

I'm thinking that's not the case but with the other movies, absolutely, there is an aesthetic that we decide would fit these movies. With *Series 7*, [a dark parody of the *Survivor* ethos] we were lampooning a genre that was shot in a specific convention—videotape. With *Chuck & Buck* it was less obvious because it was a classically composed film. For *Chuck & Buck*, Miguel wanted to work with non-professionals, which meant he probably would burn a huge amount of film, because you have to work up the performances. He wanted to create a certain aesthetic, and the tape allowed him that, while shooting freely enabled him to get the performances he got. But there's something else that happens because of the convention of video...at this point we have home video or television video, which are real, unscripted formats—news footage, or documentary footage, or home movies happening spontaneously in real time so that you don't really know what's going to happen next. You feel what is happening is more real somehow when you're looking at videotape. It's not really scripted and I think that the quality that particular convention brought to *Chuck & Buck* aided the aesthetic of the film itself. And the fact that Miguel could shoot so quickly and so lightly made it the perfect digital piece that it was.

**When *The Celebration* first came out, the distributors weren't really trumpeting its digital origins. Does digital still exude a "second class" stigma?**

When the films came up we really were not talking about the fact that they're digital. We didn't really go around saying *Chuck & Buck* was digital. But here's an amazing thing. When we sold *Chuck & Buck* to Artisan at Sundance, and we sold *Series 7* in a bidding war, no one ever said the DV word. It had nothing to do with the sale of the film. They knew we had shot it digitally but it was not a big issue; it wasn't like, "You want *how much* money for a *digital* film!?"

**Is the digital video aesthetic eroding *mise en scene*? With the ease of these small cameras, people seem to be thinking less and less about shot composition.**

I think that's a silly way of looking at it. That's like saying that you can't take a great photograph with a point-and-shoot camera. If Henri Cartier-Bresson is shooting with a point-and-shoot Nikon as opposed to his trusty Leica, he's still going to shoot beautiful photos. He's just more disciplined than the next guy. People still write beautiful novels, people still write beautiful poetry and meanwhile we all crank out pathetic emails every day in a horrible language. To me, that's just another way of saying you have no faith in artistry. *Mise en scene* involves depth of field. The fact that we have more depth of field enables us in ways to do more interesting blocking than we ever could before. *Mise en scene* doesn't mean a static camera and people walking around in it, á la Alan Resnais.

**You've said that DV has created a new language of cinema.**

I think the classically composed cinema we're used to might be less in vogue, but we'll find new forms of language. I don't think it's a lazy language, either.

If Miguel Arteta is given a digital camera, don't tell me it's not a beautifully composed film. There's laziness because of the word processor, because of the Avid, because of everything, but there are also going to be people who think in new ways because of this technology.

**Because of the technology there has been a surge of quick image captures and a dearth of slower, quieter images.**

That's valid, but then again, it is a different language.

**Those quicker shots are more indigenous to video.**

Absolutely. I think it has something to do with the randomized grain structure that is part of what gives beauty to a film. Kodak has a TMAX, which is a controlled grain structure, and then it has a PAN film, typical regular grain, which is different even on still image when you're looking at it on a film. For instance, if you take a movie like Wim Wenders' *The Goalie's Anxiety at the Penalty Kick* (1971), you have a few shots where he just cuts to a still life, because this is a movie that uses still life imagery as its leitmotif. In film, it's the background palette that changes from frame to frame, giving cinema its intrinsic poetic nature. There is an inherent fixed quality in a digital image. In video you're looking at something that's been transformed through the prism of the chip and is fixed in a certain way, and it's just not as interesting to look at.

**Do you have discussions with your filmmakers on those subjects before they shoot on video?**

We talk to them a little bit about that. On every single film we've done there's a moment where the filmmaker cuts away to something and we say, "If you were making a movie you should keep it that long, but since the origination is video, we should probably trim it because it doesn't have the same emotional effect on the audience." You have color difference—chip color is not a film color grain structure—and you have a depth of field difference too. So unless we emulate or electronically fake that stuff, we can't really achieve a filmic quality. Video will never really match that anyway, which is why it will ultimately change the language. I'm not saying it's better or worse, but the cinema that I grew up with, the quality of those images will be gone forever.

**What exactly is "circle of confusion?"**

People talk about how there is more depth of field in video. The reason is that the video chip, in relation to the lens, is a smaller image, which means technically 16mm and 8mm film have more depth of field than 35mm with the same lens. The reason is that the lens is focusing everything onto a certain plane the size of that plane. "Circle of confusion" has to do with how long the image going through the lens will be in focus as it hits the frame. What it means is, when you have a bigger image, and a bigger

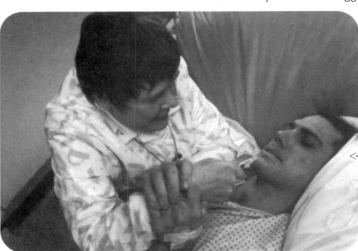

negative, an object will come out of focus faster than if you have a smaller image. Thus, you have more depth of field in video than in film.

Connie (Marylouise Burke) and Jeff (Glenn Fitzgerald) in Series 7: The Contenders .
courtesy of Blow Up Pictures/USA Films
photo by Steve Lubensky

## Will digital video kill celluloid?

Of course it will. Digital is cheaper and movies have always been too expensive. When photography was birthed in the mid-19th century, painting was hyper-realist, but as soon as a machine was invented that allowed people to record perfect images, there appeared Impressionism, Fauvism, Cubism...all those new ways of interpreting the world.

## As the theory goes: Photography freed painting and cinema freed photography. Consequently, photography has become more of a media art, and painting is considered to be an elitist enterprise. If painting, originally a widespread form of image communication, is so "free," why is it considered so "precious?" It's been completely ghettoized.

I think that will happen with true cinema. When Woody Allen chooses to make a black-and-white movie, that is a choice, and often, a more expensive choice.

## Why do filmmakers and cineastes quote Godard and Cassavetes at such an alarming rate?

The reason people reference Cassavetes for digital is very simple. He paid for his own film stock, so he shot as much as he wanted to, and the performances he got are as free as those we now get on videotape. Godard is a totally different matter: He is the pioneer of digital cinema, one of the first people to start working digitally. He made *Numero deux* on video in 1975, then moved to Tyrol [Switzerland] in 1976 and set up his own video studio. He is the Picasso of the film world. He went through every style, every format, and totally revolutionized the way we make movies.

## To you, is Dogme 95 a new wave that has brought filmmakers closer to a dialogue?

The fact is, Dogme was slightly tongue in cheek. In a way it was a PR stunt. I don't mean that in a negative way, but Dogme and digital have nothing inherently to do with each other. The intention was never to make DV features. The Dogme tenet stipulates Academy 35mm film; they stretched it to include "projected in 35mm." In a sense, Dogme was meant to be the last stand of 35mm film, which is pretty ironic.

**It certainly helped stoke the digital revolution.**

> The digital revolution is going to free up the studio system—that's how I look at it. As a production company, we can now go out and make our own movies. I can go out and buy a little camera and, for the cost of ten minutes of celluloid footage, produce an entire feature and that frees me up to make a film. I don't like video much either. It's an exciting medium, but the fact is we all hate video, and we all want to make our own work. Kodak owns our eyes, the studio owns our wallets, and the media owns everything. What used to prevent us from making films was money, but now, because of DV, we can.

**Will that bring on fresher, riskier films?**

> In the '70s, there was an intersection of art and commercial cinema, but that had to do with the studios not knowing what they should do. There was confusion at the time, and they didn't know what to greenlight and what not to. The freedom was a desperate attempt to understand the changes wrought in our culture by the revolutions of the '60s and '70s. I think we're going to see much more experimental work on one hand, and other works that will simply break through. *Blair Witch* is a good example of that—I don't think it's a good film, but it is an extraordinary one. It was made for no money, had meager distribution and became huge. Many other films came out that year, and those filmmakers complained, 'Nobody saw my film because the studios control everything.' But good or bad, *Blair Witch* proved that if you make a movie people want to see, they will find a way to see it.

## PETER BRODERICK
### Next Wave Films

Next Wave President Peter Broderick is a tireless DV booster, traveling to festivals and college campuses, winning converts with an impressive program of DV clips. Inspired by the fairy tale success of Kevin Smith's *Clerks*, Broderick launched Next Wave Films in 1997, now an arm of the Independent Film Channel. His mission? Providing finishing funds for independent films shot on film or video in the $500,000 to $3 million range, plus an array of services for ultra-low budget features from the U.S. and abroad—kind of one-stop shopping for all your indie film needs. As producer's rep, as well as sharing equity in the movie, Next Wave stipulates that their films will be shown on The Independent Film Channel when they come to basic cable.

When their theatrical distribution is over, dovetailing nicely with the business end of things, they become part of the Next Wave film library.

Broderick was not born with a Super 8 camera in hand. He graduated from Brown University with a major in American Literature before reading Economics at King's College, Cambridge University, for two years. He then went on to Yale Law School, where he also became involved in running the university's film society. While working as a public defender in Washington, DC, Broderick began writing film reviews. Soon after a fateful, three-hour interview with director Terrence Malick, he decided to quit law and pursue a film career. Broderick worked on *Days of Heaven*, and, ultimately, ran Malick's production company, Hickory Street. He has also been an active board member of both IFP/West and *Filmmaker* magazine for a number of years. Agenda 2000, the production arm of Next Wave, finances and executive produces features shot on digital video for theatrical release. Films include Kate Davis' *Southern Comfort*, Henry Barrial's *Some Body*, David and Laurie Shapiro's *Keep the River on Your Right: A Modern Cannibal Tale*, Christopher Nolan's *Following*, Joe Carnahan's *Blood, Guts, Bullets & Octane*; Jordan Melamed's *Manic* and Maxie Collier's *Paper Chasers*.

## Does DV still have an outlaw status?

There were questions about its viability that seem totally moot now. It seems to me it has become woven into the fabric of independent film. In the early- through mid-90s, the focus was how to make movies on film with smaller resources. When films like that came along they were used as models that other filmmakers could emulate. In that way Robert Rodriquez's *El Mariachi*, Kevin Smith's *Clerks*, and Nick Gomez's *Laws of Gravity* all had an outlaw status. It's always been hard for indie filmmakers to find the resources to make movies with the creative freedom they desire. Had digital been around, that would've been part of the mix.

## Have digital tools provoked a creative change in the filmmaking process?

There are things applicable to studio filmmaking that don't necessarily apply in independent filmmaking. Indie filmmaking often involves limited resources which, at the very least, guarantee that you can remain independent, but filmmakers working without corporate resources are usually obtaining them from friends and family. The idea that you can own a camera, shoot a period of time, own the editing software and use it on your computer, and that you can shoot with a 100 to one ratio, without lights, with a tiny crew in the real world is just fantastic.

**I feel that you're about to bring up Dogme 95.**

Lars von Trier has a genius for this kind of thing. Maybe it's because he used to do TV commercials. I have no idea what the truth is: My impression is that they had a half hour to kill in a pub, and they started talking and had this brainstorm which ended up being written down, but not really publicized. With the coming of [Dogme #1] *The Celebration* and [Dogme#2] *The Idiots* at Cannes it all made sense to bring it out this way. Even if those two films had shown up at the festival with no rules, they would've made an impact; but with rules, the press had a story as well.

The thing is, the press has difficulty dealing with things that are only partially true, or partially serious. Some of the Dogme rules are serious and others are almost parodies of rules. It's really hard for the press to differentiate: "Okay, rule number 7, that's a good rule. Number 5 is a mixture of both good and bad...." Nobody was going to separate it for them—what's true and what isn't—hence, the current situation.

**There was also some initial confusion about Dogme being only a DV production concept.**

Very true. When [Dogme #3] *Mifune*, which was shot on film, came out at the Berlin Film Festival, there was all this confusion about DV and film, because it was a Dogme movie and weren't Dogme movies also DV movies, and so forth. There was a rush to get tickets, and bidding for the American rights. The press was pretty excited about it. Outside of the context of Dogme, *Mifune* is a perfectly nice European art movie, but it has little to do with the spirit of Dogme. Then you look at [Dogme #4] *The King Is Alive*, and it is so different than the other two. Kristian Levring had shot commercials, but I don't think he'd ever shot digitally before. Here he is with four DV cameras in the middle of the desert—it proves you can shoot with a small format DV camera, without lighting, and create something visually quite spectacular. *The Celebration* is spectacular in its own right, but it's *cinéma vérité* spectacular. And for the actors it's such an intense experience—being accustomed to working with one camera, and suddenly not having that restriction. They were able to perform in an open space, to get what was needed under highly adverse circumstance, and still get this visual knockout.

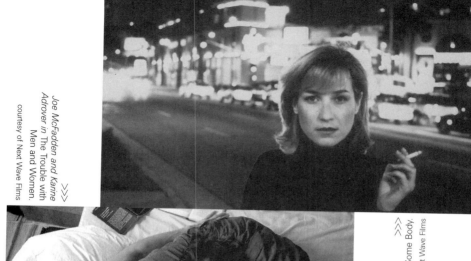

**It makes you realize that the spirit of Dogme
encompasses a fairly wide canvas.**

And it takes things in a reinvigorating new direction. But von
Trier is a filmmaker who is continually taking risks. You can say
his first couple of movies had a common style, but since *Breaking
the Waves*, each thing has been very different than the thing
before. Alfred Hitchcock, John Ford—they had a style and way of
working that was constantly being refined and perfected; but how
many filmmakers are there in the world who take real chances,
who are continually reinventing themselves and the way they
work? I would also count Mike Figgis in that category.

**What about DV filmmaking being reinvented
in some quarters as simply a way to make
cheap movies?**

To those who say that DV just means more bad movies, I say that
if we haven't drowned in a sea of Hollywood mediocrity yet, I
doubt we'll drown in a sea of digital mediocrity now. But the

economics of filmmaking are fundamental—you can't separate them from the creative or economic side. Production companies everywhere are starting digital divisions and their objective is to make more movies for less money. But the Hollywood studio system is not about making movies for less money, so if we begin to see digital features being made at the studio level, they will probably have higher budgets.

## Will independent filmmakers more and more turn to DV?

A number of filmmakers will always believe that they can only do what they want to do on 35mm. Many will be interested in combining the two. Newer filmmakers who don't have as much of a history with the film medium will naturally gravitate towards DV, but the established, experienced filmmakers are at least as enthusiastic, if not more so, about DV. They completely understand; the genie is out of the bottle and it's not going back in. Spike Lee...I heard him say, on a panel in Cannes in May, 1999, that he "wasn't the least bit interested in shooting with digital." In September of that same year, he went into production with his first DV film, *Bamboozled.*

## The quality achievable in a DV-to-film transfer is improving all the time.

As well as the cameras themselves. I've seen a number of things where you couldn't tell that it didn't originate on 35mm. For instance, von Trier's *Dancer in the Dark.* When it premiered at Cannes, most thought it was shot on film, but not one second of that movie originated on film.

## Do you think digital tools are shifting power from financiers to filmmakers?

Absolutely. In the old studio system, it can be three years between movies. Now, we can use the resources we have or get, which includes cast, crew, camera. You can make a movie a year if you want. You don't need to spend time raising money, so you can be committed to making the movie itself; and when it comes to distribution, digital projectors will help. That means we won't have to worry about raising $40,000 or $50,000 before Sundance for a 35mm transfer. You can screen it at a festival, and if the enthusiasm is there, it becomes easier to find the funds for that transfer. And, if the enthusiasm isn't there, it can still be shown on television, broadcast satellite, or home video.

## You're not convinced that the Internet is a viable distribution system?

The quality is still crappy. If you want to watch three minutes of a high concept short, maybe, but we've really got to come up with a whole new level of delivery. Less than 50 percent of American homes have Internet access, and most of those have it at 28.8. A sliver of the population has DSL. I have a state-of-the-art computer, but when I try to download I still get kind of a freeze frame for about thirty seconds, where I can hear the audio, but no active picture, then I get two frames a second, then back to freeze frame. It's unbearable even for a four-minute movie. So I'm saying, let's be realistic: It's not happening now, and it may not be that much better in the next couple of years.

## Even so, there is such passion at the grassroots level for neophyte filmmakers.

Maybe it's the times we live in; the Internet is perceived as being very glamorous. If you look at the history, from the late '70s to the early '90s, and you think about the most talented filmmakers that emerged then, you think of John Sayles, Spike Lee, David Lynch, Gus Van Sant, Wayne Wang, Jim Jarmusch. They all started out at the grassroots level, making pretty low budget movies—but they were expecting to make their movies that way, whereas others were trying to raise that first million for a first feature. The filmmakers I mentioned are all still making movies today, and when they started, were determined to make movies despite the economics of production. Having demonstrated their talents, they could move on and up, and it became easier to get resources after that, but for a lot of people it was too intimidating. You had to know people, you had to network, and you needed to attend the right schools so you could network with the right people.

## With DV breaking down rules and barriers in filmmaking, do you think that will impact cinema's timeworn gender barrier?

It's still an old boy network, but now that you have the opportunity to make a film for $1,000, you don't need to be in the old boy network to access the resources. The percentage of women behind the camera is depressing, at least in the movies we are receiving. We got 500 movies from around the world last year and, even though women outnumber men on the planet, many more men than women are making movies. I hope to see some fabulous new films from women that will inspire other women to make movies.

## How do you decide which movies you want to take on?

Within a few minutes of watching, I can tell if a filmmaker has got it, and that he or she will be making a lot of terrific movies for years to come. That's quite apart from the success of failure of an individual movie. For me, what it comes down to with film-makers is their visual sense, their ability to work with actors to create characters, and to create an energy in the way the story is told. It's what I often say in my presentations: There is only one reason to be an independent filmmaker, and the reason is quite simple. It's because you have no choice. If it's not total compulsion, it doesn't make sense.

## Do you ever feel more like a mentor than a film producer?

There is certainly a Johnny Appleseed quality to the job. I have the chance to support individual, iconic filmmakers who have a passion for filmmaking. I never thought of it this way before, but it's kind of like being a simultaneous translator, in that I understand things about DV filmmaking, but I can also communicate with people in the "analog" world. I feel very lucky in what I'm doing. I'm living in a moment in history where filmmaking is changing, changing in a revolutionary way. For me it's not a job, it's a mission—a very fun mission.

## SCOTT MACAULAY
### Forensic Films

Columbia University graduate Scott Macaulay, and his Forensic partner-in-crime, Robin O'Hara, met in New York, in the mid-80s at the experimental performance space The Kitchen. O'Hara was the head of the video distribution program and Macaulay was the programming director. Taking over from previous curator/performer Eric Bogosian [Talk Radio], he developed all the performance and theater work for the arts collective for seven years.

In 1989, James Schamus [Good Machine] asked Macaulay to come on as associate producer for Raoul Ruiz's The Golden Boat (1990). He and Forensic have since produced Tom Noonan's two films What Happened Was... (1994) and The

*Wife* (1996); Frank Whaley's *Joe the King* (1999), Harmony Korine's *Gummo* (1997) and *julien donkey-boy* [1999]; Jessie Peretz's *First Love, Last Rites* (1997) and *The Chateau* (2001), amongst others.

Macaulay, who still resides in New York, is also one of the founders of *Filmmaker* magazine.

## You began as a programmer at Manhattan's experimental performance space, The Kitchen?

My partner Robin O'Hara and I met at the Kitchen. Robin was the head of the video distribution program; I was the programming director and curated all the performance and theater work. I worked there for seven years—right after Eric Bogosian [*Talk Radio*]. I did film work, curatorially, at Columbia University, then moved into live performance after college, but I always intended to get back into film.

## You are also still working with founders of *Filmmaker* magazine?

I've been with *Filmmaker* since the beginning, and, although it's a quarterly, it's still a bit of a juggling act.

## How did you become interested in producing DV films?

I wasn't, until I worked at The Kitchen as a programmer. I was the development director, which meant I was in charge of fundraising. My particular fundraising forte was government funds—National Endowment of the Arts (NEA), New York State Council on the Arts (NYSCA)—and at that time there was a strict division between film and video. They were entirely separate media. There were aesthetic issues at work but there were also historical, bureaucratic and administrative issues in the way the funding bodies dealt with the different media. The Kitchen was slightly attacked for blending the two. When Amy Taubin [film critic for the *Village Voice*] was selected as curator in the late-80s she was someone who came from film, and the video community was temporarily affronted.

## It was Good Machine's James Schamus who kick-started you into your new career, wasn't it?

It was around 1989, before Schamus [the producer/writer of *Crouching Tiger, Hidden Dragon*] formed Good Machine with Ted Hope. We were both on the boards of theater companies: I was with the Squat Theater and he was working with the Wooster

Group. One day he called me up and said "Do you want to help
me produce a film by by Raoul Ruiz, *The Golden Boat*? He's this
great Chilean director." Ruiz was teaching at Harvard and James
had an idea to make a film with him over three long weekends in
January. I asked, "Do you have any money?" He said, "No, but
we'll get it." I said, "It's October now...." "Yeah, yeah—do you
want to do it?" Robin and I did, so I was the associate producer,
Robin was the production manager, Christine Vachon was first
AD and Maryse Alberti shot it.

**Some very interesting people worked on
that shoot.**

They were people I'd worked with in the performance world, like
Kathy Acker and Annie Sprinkle [stripper/performance artist],
people from Squat Theater, and Vito Acconci were all in the
film. That was kind of my first film experience.

**So, you left The Kitchen and took the plunge
into filmmaking?**

I was also working as a part-time reader for New Line Cinema,
so they recommended me for a producing fellowship at
Sundance. I got the fellowship and the first movie that we produced was Tom Noonan's *What Happened Was...* (1994), which came
out of a little bit of development work I was doing for Good
Machine at the time. After discovering Tom as a writer and seeing his play, basically Ted Hope from Good Machine said, "If
you and Robin can commit to producing it, we'll come up with
a free camera for you, and Tom has $50,000." We shot it in
September 1992, and it wound up premiering at Sundance in
1994. We formed Forensic a couple of years later.

I think in my head I knew the video world so well, whether it
was commercial or pure video art like Naim June Paik or Bill
Viola. I think that having worked in that environment, absorb-
ing those distinctions between video and film made me more
cautious in terms of accepting video as a form that will be accepted in the film world. That's why doing Harmony Korine's first
digital feature, *julien donkey-boy* (1999) was interesting. It was the
first thing we did on video, although Robin had produced
Michael Almereyda's short (*Another Girl Another Planet*), in
PXLvision, but that had a more experimental intent.

## How did you end up as one of the producers of *julien donkey-boy*?

The short version of the story is that Cary Woods [Independent Pictures] had his production company set up at Miramax. Miramax was very impressed with how *Kids* had done, and they were very interested in doing something with Cary. The fact that Harmony's agent [John Lescher] was negotiating *Boogie Nights* at the same time for Paul Thomas Anderson didn't hurt either. It was a combination of things.

In 1997 we'd done Harmony's *Gummo* [financed by New Line, shot by Jean Yves Escoffier in 35mm] together so the relationship with Harmony was already there, but the roots of *julien* are really in *Gummo*. That was Harmony's first film and he had a lot of ideas and ways that he wanted to approach filmmaking, which, in many cases, we were able to realize. Harmony is somebody who embraces spontaneity: The paradox is that he's an extremely good writer, but he's also the first person to abandon

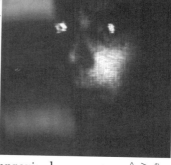

*Ewen Bremner in* julien donkey-boy
<< photo by Anthony Dod Mantle

the script for a totally unscripted and improvised moment, or to adapt something for a particular location. In that shopping mall scene where they're handing out leaflets looking for the cat, that's entirely filmed with a hidden 35mm camera. But there were moments like that that Harmony really wanted but were difficult to do with 35mm. When I saw the first cut of *Gummo*, I was shocked at all the video material in the film, because none of that material was shot during production, or very little of it. It was stuff that Harmony had: little video clips from television or taken at friends' houses. Most of that stuff was shot during the location scouting a month or two before the shoot began.

## So, you're looking at the first edit...

It was like, "Where did *this* stuff come from? Who *are* these people?" It was a legal nightmare because we had no release forms; we had to do video stills of them and canvass the neighborhood and track them all down. That was really the start of Harmony's interest in video, and in the texture of video in that film. All that video was photographed by the DP—off a monitor—but with different distances between the camera and the monitor, and pushed to accentuate the video line. Some of the video Harmony had was crummy VHS with roll bars, too.

After *Gummo*, he was trying to decide what to do next. I'd written something for *Dazed and Confused* [magazine] about DYI filmmaking—people shooting things on video and editing on desktops—which Harmony read and liked. So he called up and said, "It's funny you wrote this piece because I'm also working on something that is going to be done entirely on video, and I want to do it in a totally different way." He had a very loose treatment, twenty pages, sixty or seventy scenes, no dialogue, improvisation, with surveillance camera aesthetics. Taking things that he did in *Gummo*, and doing it so much more in the film. By this time he'd seen *Celebration* and was inspired by that and very interested in working with its DP, Anthony Dod Mantle. It also struck me as being realistic from a production point of view to do some of what he wanted to do using these small cameras. If it was a full 35mm setup we wouldn't be able to maintain those aspects of mobility. Doing it Dogme style was decided upon very close to the shooting. As to Harmony "breaking the rules"...he had written the treatment before it became a Dogme film, and when it became a Dogme film, he didn't want to change it. All I can really say is that there is nothing depicted that is fake. In that scene where you see Julien [the actor Ewen Bremner] throttling the kid, it's entirely from the point of view of the kid's eyeglass cameras. Then you see Julien burying something, but you don't know what it is—and by the way, under the Dogme standards, there is no "fake" simulation of a murder. It's all suggested.

### Why are so many people inspired by *Celebration*?

Its shooting and cutting style seems very fresh. The story is strong, funny and dramatic, and there is no technological theme to the story. Only in the deepest kind of subtextual level of the film, in the decay of the social structure.

### What's your take on digital video production nowadays?

You go and see something like *Chuck & Buck*, which is a very intimate character based movie, and I think that my thinking has evolved. As cameras and transfers get better, I think that the medium can encompasses these other types of stories.

**Your interest is the medium has clearly grown.**
*The Chateau* **(2001) was also shot on video.**

Yes, with the director Jessie Peretz, whom we worked with on *First Love, Last Rites* (1997). Like *julien, The Chateau* was also improvised, but with more of a treatment and no actual script. It is much more linear and straightforward story, about two American brothers who unexpectedly inherit a Chateau in the South of France. A few years ago I would've said no to doing this project on video.

It came about because Jessie, Robin and I were having dinner and we and a couple of other people were developing two screenplays for him, slightly bigger movies. Jesse was originally very anti-video, but the scripts were taking a long time to get finished and everyone was sort of frustrated. I said that we should find a way to do something quickly, something small that we could finance easily. I always had this romantic idea of the kind of movie where you get a bunch of actors and go to some distant location. One of the people at the dinner brought up the Chateau idea, and by the end of the meal we had a first act of what would happen with these characters. Everyone traded ideas back and forth for a month. Robin took all the ideas one day and assembled them into an outline and threw a couple of new ideas in the mix, and then we tried to get money for it. We had it budgeted at $700,000, but everyone said we can't give you money without a script.

We approached Dolly Hall [producer of *johns* (1996)] who was then at the digital division at [production company] Greenestreet. She said, "If you can do it at $250,000, we can find a way, but we can't do it at this level." So we went back and retooled the whole thing and re-envisioned it as more of a no-budget film, got money from them and another investor, called Crossroads, and came up with this plan to shoot this movie in twelve days. Honestly, we were very surprised at the level of actors we were able to get with this very slender idea. Paul Rudd had seen *Celebration*, and even though ours wasn't a Dogme film, everyone was excited by that kind of approach.

Our DP, Tom Richmond (*Little Odessa* [1994]), shot in fourteen days, using PAL [European format] Sony TRV 900, the

*Chloe Sevigny in* julien donkey-boy
photo by Anthony Dod Mantle

same camera as *julien*, just because we had two of them. Gaspar Noe [the director of *I Stand Alone* (1998)], who lives in Paris, is a friend and he recommended his grip and electric crew and his AD. Although it ended up costing around $300,000, it all came together—but Jesse told me, "It wasn't until the third day of shooting I thought this project could work."

**Even so, versus film, there was a real savings in the budget.**

Absolutely. On a low budget film, film stock is always a huge conflict between the producer and the director. But the savings are not just in stock but being able to work with smaller crews, and you can work non-union easier. You might not need a Teamster, or not as many Teamsters.

**Are you getting a lot of calls from people who want you to finance their films on video?**

Yeah, and it can be kind of overwhelming. People are overly concerned about the technical issues, whereas it really should be more like, "Hey, is this project really applicable to digital, is this a good plan?" I shot this film called *Chasing Sleep* right before Jesse's film. We did that one on 35mm. That was a good plan.

# Dogme95 and the New Guard

*I had better start this whole thing on an optimistic note. Pessimists never discover much, and to find a whole universe (what a tall order!), you've got to be looking around open-mindedly.*

*So I hope my very optimistic approach is not going to shock you.*

*It starts with the following thesis:*

*The future of the cinema no longer lies in its past.*

*Or the other way around: The past of the cinema will not help us much to lead us into its future. "Hey, what's so very optimistic about that?" some of you might say. "We've learned*

## Wim Wenders

### germany
### WHAT THE NEW
### TECHNOLOGIES OFFER

*everything we know about the cinema from its past. It's dear to us! We're good at what we know from it! Why wouldn't that knowledge carry us—and our cinema—into the future? This guy sounds more like a pessimist."*

*I am not. I fully and totally believe in the future of the cinema, and especially our European one, more than ever. I love and cherish its history.*

But I have lost all confidence whatsoever in nostalgia. The future of the cinema is just about to get invented, and its past is no longer the obvious bridge into what is about to come. Why? I believe that the digital revolution, of which we are witnessing but the first phase for the last few years, is not that much based on evolution as we all might like to believe. I have the impression it's rather reconstructing cinema from scratch.

When sound came up, some seventy years ago, a lot of rules changed while some stayed the same. Films looked less elegant for a while, certainly, and the elaborate language of the silent era was reduced and crippled at first. But not for that long: Film incorporated the new technology of sound pretty fast, recovered and grew and became more complex than ever.

The "new technologies" however are not just an extension of film, even if they introduced themselves as such at first. They don't just add a dimension, the way sound did. They will not be incorporated; rather, they are taking over. They are about to replace "film."

I am not just referring to the material, to celluloid. I am referring to everything you and I know about our craft, our art, our industry. The entire landscape of film is about to be shaken up completely. Its past will no longer be its future....

Don't worry: I suppose we will all continue to do what we do: We will be actors, directors, producers, writers, cameramen, agents, set designers, editors, composers and so on.

The entire landscape of film is about to be shaken up COMPLETELY.

Its past will no longer be its future....

We will all continue to work in that large field of storytelling, in the realm of the audio-visual world. Our profession might even continue to be called "Filmmaking."

But it won't be based on what we know now or what we've learned from the past.

I don't pretend to know more than you. I have worked a bit inside that new digital world; I have learned how to use the new tools, just a bit; I have made some music videos and commercials; I have shot on virtual sets; I have worked in High-Definition; shot two entire films digitally; done some special-effects work; sat on machines like the Henry, the Flame, the Inferno; worked on the Fire, the C-Reality, just enough to understand that I have only opened a door and taken a peek into a new landscape. I feel like the guy in that famous drawing from the Middle Ages who breaks through the skin that is wrapped around the Earth and sees the planets and the stars out there, in amazement. I feel like I want to turn around and tell you that the Earth is not flat. It's really in those dimensions that I see the impact of the so-called new technologies: Cinema is not flat, and we don't have an idea yet what's out there.

Even Lars von Trier with his historical step into this future (I'm talking about Dancer in the Dark), even Tom Tykwer with Run Lola Run, even Luc Besson, even Steven Spielberg, George Lucas, Roland Emmerich and with them other directors who have faced and embraced the new technologies—even they don't know all that much about the vast open territory in front of us.

Right now filmmaking seems to me to be at the age when the first scientists imagined nuclear energy and then eventually managed to split matter for the first time. Little did they know. It's like that now. We have just learned how each image and each sound can be split up down to its atoms and be put back together. But we are still handling those images with the same narrative structures, the same dramaturgy, the same storytelling recipes, the same storyboards and editing techniques used by Griffith, Chaplin or Abel Gance. Basically.

We can feed film into computers so that it becomes immaterial information, of which every bit, every single atom, can be worked at, manipulated, changed and replaced. Then we can output the result back to film, as if nothing ever happened. But we have not changed all the tools around. We're still toying around with a new nuclear technology of images but have no clue where it is taking us.

You see, that's why I'm an optimist. Because I imagine the future of storytelling, where directors, writers, producers, actors, cameramen, etc., actually start controlling that nuclear technology that we will have at our disposal, not just playing around with it.

feelings…nothing other than the human mind and the human heart.

Digital technology doesn't do that. It doesn't do anything on its own.

Technology is not entertaining us, not teaching us, not moving us. In the future of cinema you still have to do that.

You know what word I hate most today? "Content."

It comes out of a very insecure time of transition in which technology rules. We can do so much, all of a sudden, that this new digital technology of transmission is encouraged and pretends to be the essential thing itself, so that what it transports is only of secondary nature, only "content."

Can you feel how condescending that word is?

I am looking forward to the future where technology will be so boring again that the only exciting thing will be, once more, what you say with it, what you express with it.

Mind you, I am not talking against the new technologies now. In the very contrary:

I rather suggest accepting it as given that they are here to stay and to change the cinema. But I would like to encourage you to imagine how to overcome that situation of imbalance between technology and "content."

We're still toying around
with a new nuclear technology of images
but HAVE NO CLUE where it is taking us.

I'd be happy if that would still be called filmmaking. Although that doesn't really matter. What we do with all the new toys—that is what matters. Technologies never do anything you don't make them do. Nothing else produces poetry, beauty, truth, drama, tension or human

If the biggest advertising factor for a film today is its special effects, meaning the mere technology used to tell a story, and if the story and the characters play second fiddle to these effects, then we are in the process of giving up our craft to our tools.

Already today it is getting difficult to get a wide release for a film in the U.S. (still the biggest market for films in the world) unless you make extensive use of digital effects. Distributors are simply not interested in your "product."

And that is a phenomenon that we will face in Europe soon as well.

I see a generation of moviegoers and film-freaks growing up for whom effects are already more important than storylines, who already confuse motion with emotion.

Again, I am not complaining here. On the contrary. I can't accept to look at that situation from a position of "victimisation." There is a much better attitude!

Which is: We have to master that nuclear technology.

We have to learn how to use it.

Right now it is, in effect, starting to use us.

We have to embrace the New Technologies in a big way.

We have to make sure that we learn to master them, that a new generation of filmmakers has access to all of it.

There is nothing right now that can be done in Hollywood, that could not be done in Paris or London or Munich or Barcelona or anywhere else in Europe. We have great post-production facilities here in Europe. A lot of the future software is developed here or in Asia.

We are in a good position here in Europe.

European cinema is a huge, endless fountain of creativity, of fantasy and of imagination.

We are backed up by the longest tradition of theater, literature, painting, poetry, architecture, music—everything that can help to turn cold digital technology into an emotional new language of cinema.

In a few years, there will be data beamers standing next to the good old movie projectors, and in another few years, those projectors will be gone. The entire history of cinema will be available in any theater via servers, optical cables, satellites,

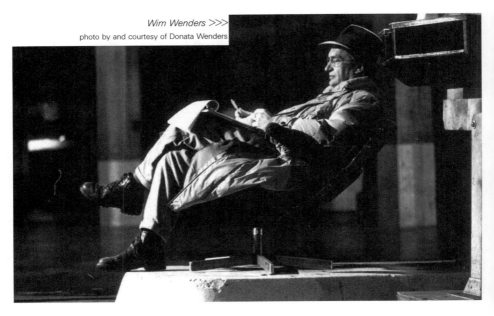

Wim Wenders >>>
photo by and courtesy of Donata Wenders

broadband or whatever system. We want to make sure that this important transformation happens in our control, that the norms regulating this giant change do not exclude us and won't be dictated by others. Whoever finances the huge cost of installing these new facilities in cinemas all over Europe will also control the programming. Let's make sure that we are not at the short end of this development.

The future of the European Cinema might not be as much based on its past, as we all would like to believe, and that is okay, as long as we have confidence that the future remains to be invented.

Right now it might seem to many, as if all that digital technology was invented mainly to blow things up and to create new and cheaper ways to depict destruction, all sorts of horror and brutality.

It would be so very nearsighted to constrain it to that.

It would be fatal to fold our hands and say: "We can't beat that!"

To say, "We don't want to work with these tools."

It is up to us and to the next generation of talent here in Europe to put the new digital technologies into the service of all sorts of storytelling and push them into realms nobody has opened up yet.

Only this technology will help us to explore new territories of storytelling, adequate to grasp the reality of the 21st century.

We can't make new expeditions into the human mind and the human heart with the hardware of the 19th century.

This cinema of the future does not yet exist. We see glimpses of it, glimpses of an incredible richness of expression. And that is my optimistic outlook, my introduction to our "boat ride" today.

Technology can't do anything on its own. You have to force it to start swinging, maybe even dancing. (Otherwise we'll all end up as dancers

**We can't make new EXPEDITIONS into the human MIND and the human HEART with the hardware of the 19th century.**

in the dark.) The power, the poetry and the imagination are only in the hands of people who have learned to use their tools. There is an abundance of new tools just lying around.

We have to start shaping the future cinema with them.

# THE MANIFESTO

**DOGME 95**... is a collective of film directors founded in Copenhagen in spring 1995.

DOGME 95 has the expressed goal of countering "certain tendencies" in the cinema today.

**DOGME 95 is a rescue action!**

In 1960 enough was enough! The movie was dead and called for resurrection. The goal was correct but the means were not! The New Wave proved to be a ripple that washed ashore and turned to muck.

Slogans of individualism and freedom created works for a while, but no changes. The wave was up for grabs, like the directors themselves. The wave was never stronger than the men behind it. The anti-bourgeois cinema itself became bourgeois, because the foundations upon which its theories were based was the bourgeois perception of art. The auteur concept was bourgeois romanticism from the very start and thereby—false!

To DOGME 95 cinema is not individual!

Today a technological storm is raging, the result of which will be the ultimate democratisation of the cinema. For the first time, anyone can make movies. But the more accessible the media becomes, the more important the avant-garde. It is no accident that the phrase "avant-garde" has military connotations. Discipline is the answer...we must put our films into uniform, because the individual film will be decadent by definition!

DOGME 95 counters the individual film by the principle of presenting an indisputable set of rules known as THE VOW OF CHASTITY.

In 1960 enough was enough! The movie had been cosmeticised to death, they said; yet since then the use of cosmetics has exploded.

The "supreme" task of the decadent filmmakers is to fool the audience. Is that what we are so proud of? Is that what the "100 years" have brought us? Illusions via which emotions can be communicated? By the individual artist's free choice of trickery?

Predictability (dramaturgy) has become the golden calf around which we dance. Having the characters' inner lives justify the plot is too complicated, and not "high art." As never before, the superficial action and the superficial movie are receiving all the praise.

The result is barren. An illusion of pathos and an illusion of love.

To DOGME 95 the movie is not illusion!

Today a technological storm is raging of which the result is the elevation of cosmetics to God. By using new technology anyone at any time can wash the last grains of truth away in the deadly embrace of sensation. The illusions are everything the movie can hide behind.

DOGME 95 counters the film of illusion by the presentation of an indisputable set of rules known as THE VOW OF CHASTITY.

## THE VOW OF CHASTITY

"I swear to submit to the following set of rules drawn up and confirmed by DOGME 95:

1. Shooting must be done on location. Props and sets must not be brought in (if a particular prop is necessary for the story, a location must be chosen where this prop is to be found).
2. The sound must never be produced apart from the images or vice versa. (Music must not be used unless it occurs where the scene is being shot).
3. The camera must be handheld. Any movement or immobility attainable in the hand is permitted. (The film must not take place where the camera is standing; shooting must take place where the film takes place).
4. The film must be in color. Special lighting is not acceptable. (If there is too little light for exposure the scene must be cut or a single lamp be attached to the camera).
5. Optical work and filters are forbidden.
6. The film must not contain superficial action. (Murders, weapons, etc. must not occur.)
7. Temporal and geographical alienation are forbidden. (That is to say that the film takes place here and now.)
8. Genre movies are not acceptable.
9. The film format must be Academy 35 mm.
10. The director must not be credited.

Furthermore I swear as a director to refrain from personal taste! I am no longer an artist. I swear to refrain from creating a "work," as I regard the instant as more important than the whole. My supreme goal is to force the truth out of my characters and settings. I swear to do so by all the means available and at the cost of any good taste and any aesthetic considerations.

Thus I make my VOW OF CHASTITY."

Copenhagen, Monday 13 March 1995

On behalf of DOGME 95

Lars von Trier        Thomas Vinterberg

# THE MEN WHO WOULD BE DOGME

"Hey Dogme boy!" calls out a cheery voice, likely a fan or a friend, but Harmony Korine can't stop, can't slow down. Already in motion, the shaggy-haired twenty-seven-year-old filmmaker, a self-proclaimed arch-terrorist of the Hollywood dream-factory, and current messenger of *julien donkey-boy*, the first American film to be birthed from the controversial cinematic strictures of the Dogme 95 manifesto, is striding confidently out of the crowded New York Film Festival press conference that followed the screening. He takes a cheeky, over-the-shoulder glance at the receding press corps, the approving applause and loud conversation, and murmurs into my ear, "You know what's so funny? When people asked me questions, I used to lie, I used to make up things all the time." Moving toward the exit, pulling out a beat up pack of cigarettes, he adds, "But I found that after Dogme 95, telling the truth could be even more shocking."

Even before *julien* achieved critical mass, Korine's highly developed sense of provocation had already inflamed the early days of his career, which began when he dropped out of NYU, scripted Larry Clark's *Kids* (at nineteen), and then wrote and directed his own feature *Gummo*, a surrealistic tale of two backwoods cat killers, which two years later managed to engender the love of filmmakers Bernardo Bertolucci and Werner Herzog, as well as the steely distemper of a New York Times critic, who called it the "worst film of the year."

Unsquelched, Korine had long been formulating *julien*, a film based on his schizophrenic Uncle Eddie, who is a permanent patient at Creedmore Psychiatric Center in Queens. Looking for a new form of high profile, low budget expression, he had been gearing up to shoot the project on digital video, and before choosing Ewen Bremner (who brilliantly constructed the layers of his character by listening to audio tapes of Eddie and by working for several months at New York's Wards Island for the Criminally Insane) had initially thought of casting himself, or his Uncle, or perhaps some other available, un-camera shy schizophrenic in the title role. One month away from production, recalls Korine, he received his next glowing neon on-ramp to viable anarchy via an enticing call from *Breaking the Waves'* mercurial director Lars von Trier.

Along with fellow Danish directors Thomas Vinterberg, Søren Kragh-Jacobsen and Kristian Levring, the collective had caused a firestorm in film circles with their Dogme 95 manifesto, a stripped-down production concept promulgated in conjunction with the high-profile 1998 Cannes premieres of the first two Dogme films: Vinterberg's award-winning, incestuous family drama, *The Celebration*; and von Trier's corrosively funny view of the bourgeoisie, *The Idiots*, which caused a massive censorship imbroglio as it contains a full-on orgy, including a twenty-second gang-bang, complete with erect penises and actual penetration. (Ironically, it never raised an eyebrow in Denmark, which abolished the censor in 1969).

In a tenderly ironic juxtaposition, the doctrine's monastic, technology-reactive rule system, to which all Dogme films must adhere, was heralded as a "Vow of Chastity." Reading like a cross between the ten commandments and an anarchist pamphlet, the ten-point plan dictates the use of handheld cameras and location shooting, and prohibits production design, props, soundtrack scores, optical work, genre storylines and—toppling decades of possessive credit wrangling—specifically eschews onscreen directorial credit.

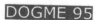

Sensing some heavy-duty running with the indie-film wolves, Korine instantly, eagerly, took von Trier up on his Dogmetic proposition. Despite the severe rule breaking which came after, for which he has been roundly chastised (and has made penance for by confession, which all the brethren's filmmakers are bound to should there be any transgression), he says the strictures of the process forced his usual haphazard bravura into a different mode of creation. "It's what Lars says. The more you restrict yourself the more freedom you get. That's the paradox. When I stuck these ten Dogme rules up on the wall, and worked within

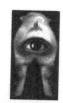

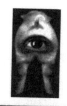

that context, I couldn't hide behind anything. When I followed them, it became a kind of wonderful, blind faith. Now," he says mournfully, a mist of gray, iridescent cigarette smoke forming above his head, "I wish I could stop with the cigarettes. Maybe I could get some more rules from my Danish film brothers."

"One piece of advice when you see him," he drawls. "Don't play pinball with him. He really likes to win."

Regarded as one of Europe's most iconoclastic, principled auteurs (with all the old school honor that bestows), von Trier has had every one of his feature films appear in the official program at Cannes, from his 1984 debut, *Element of Crime*, through 1987's *Epidemic*, 1991's *Europa* (U.S. title, *Zentropa*), and the harrowing *Breaking the Waves*, winner of the Grand Prix in 1996. One of von Trier's celebrated phobias precludes him from flying, so when he does travel, it's rarely far from the suburban Copenhagen home where he was born, and has lived off and on his entire life; a stone's throw away from the new home he now shares with his second wife Bente and their young twin sons.

Notoriously moody and wary of outsiders, von Trier likes to make an appearance on his own terms and in his own good time. I haven't seen him in over a year, following the Danish premiere of *The Idiots*, where he arrived somewhat stiffly dressed in a tuxedo, one eye on the theater EXIT signs. We're meeting at Zentropa, which in the past eight years has emerged as one of the most successful film and television production companies in Scandinavia. Recently relocated to an isolated centerpoint between the Copenhagen airport and its former quarters in the center of town, the sprawling complex previously served as the site of an old military barracks. The faceless buildings now house production offices, editing bays, soundstages and all the typical tools of a Hollywood studio. The relaxed employees wandering the grounds look like stunningly healthy recruits from a J. Crew catalogue.

Von Trier is a coolly perceptive man in his forties, of average height, with watchful, almond shaped eyes and a newly shorn head, a renewal ritual he sometimes performs at the end of a film shoot. Today he is dressed casually in comfortable pants and sandals over socks. Nodding a relaxed hello, he turns and motions for me to follow him to his small army-style jeep. Sitting down in the driver's seat, he flexes his arm up and down, and mentions he has just come from a successful two-hour tennis game, where he trounced his opponent. He smiles. "Perhaps you'd like to play?"

With Cannes 2000, and his Palme d'Or winning *Dancer in the Dark* behind him, von Trier is ready to talk about his $15 million feature, featuring French cinema-icon Catherine Denueve, with music composed by and starring Iceland's moody pop-chanteuse Björk, and in part about an Eastern European woman who imagines America as one big movie musical. It is rumored that 100 digital cameras were used during the dancing sequences. "I'm sorry, I can't talk to you about her," he answers in his softly accented English. "I promised Björk I wouldn't talk about working with her." But von Trier, who loves to sing, does say he co-wrote the lyrics for the film with Björk's music partner, Sigurjon B. Sigurdsson. Though it's clouding up, the norm for this time of year, von Trier remarks on what an extraordinarily beautiful summer it's been. "Next week," he announces, with a happy sigh, "I am going to Jutland for four days. Fly fishing. Me alone. No one. Just me."

He parks the jeep in front of his bungalow. "I chose this one, because this is the one where they originally kept the ammunition. The bunkers around it are designed so if somehow the ammunition exploded it would not destroy the whole camp. The pressure would go straight up and not out." He says this with all the wide-eyed faith of a teenager with his first science kit, adding, "I thought it would be very good, if my creative kind of power became too strong."

Inside the airy space there are all the varied comforts of home: a white shag rug, a large, comfortable couch, a refrigerator stocked with vodka and champagne, a massive TV set and a gorgeous, mint condition *Raiders of the Lost Ark* pinball machine. Von Trier sees me staring at it. "Would you like to play this?" he asks, his face lighting up. I mention Korine and von Trier laughs, and indicates the scattered mountain of video cassettes in front of the monitor. He points to one, a video of *julien,* and says, "That Harmony is a completely crazy guy. That's good. That's just what we need." Though he takes no refreshment himself, he presses a paper cup into my hands containing a very hospitable shot of Jack Daniels, adding encouragingly, "I'm for the craziness."

As are all the Dogme brothers. Crazy behavior has powerfully moving results. As Vinterberg pointed out modestly about his own *Celebration,* "I was told that two people who saw the film fainted. After they recovered, they went back and saw the rest of the film. I know it might sound a bit sadistic, but that was a huge compliment." As incest, infidelity and racism figure heavily in his tale of a family gathered together to celebrate their father's sixtieth birthday, Vinterberg says many people want to know if it's based on personal experience. "Most of it came from my imagination, I swear! My own family, I promise you, is very lovable. Although I don't know what they would've done if I'd suddenly wept and confessed, 'Yes, yes, that is me.'"

Birthing the Dogme 95 manifesto, says von Trier, has caused him great joy, as well as massive stress. Four years ago, struggling with the creative soul-searching *Breaking the Waves* brought him, he rang up Vinterberg and the two sat down, and "amongst much mirth, which went hand in hand with complete seriousness," discussed everything they mutually loathed about the conventions of commercial filmmaking. They then forbade each action one by one until, in around a half an hour, the rules took shape. As the concept mushroomed into the hot new discourse in international film circles, calls began flooding in asking for a policing of stricter interpretations, asking the King of Dogme to set the record straight.

"I don't want to be the King anymore! Please, take the mantle... I...we...are just figuring all this out now. Yes, it is COMPLETELY serious to me, it's *Wonderful,* but I can't...ach... this stupid brotherhood. This is what happens when you form a collective!"

In light of this, the four Danes recently released a joint statement, backing Korine's multi-rule breaking *julien* as a Dogme film, as well as describing the ensuing creation of a secretariat that would deal with such concerns. The most recent word is that they've decided to amend their previous method of certification of films made according to the 1995 manifesto. If a filmmaker feels that his film applies, he may send a sworn declaration stating that he followed the rules to the Dogme secretariat, and a couple of weeks later he will receive the Dogme 95 certificate. Filmmakers can cheat, but, the logic goes, they'll only be cheating themselves.

The manifesto was never intended to be a fashionable cloak to hide behind, says von Trier. That would be pointless.

"Please, take the mantle," von Trier implores. He clamps his hand over his eyes and leans into the couch. "I don't want to be the King anymore! Please, take the mantle. I just want to go fly fishing. I know, I don't know, I don't know. Don't ask me to answer these questions. I...we...are just figuring all this out now. Yes, it is completely serious to me, it's wonderful, but I can't...ach...this stupid brotherhood. This is what happens when you form a collective!"

Vinterberg, 31, whose talent, charm and good looks make him a poster-boy for the beneficial effects of Dogme living, says he took up the challenge because he felt stuck with a lot of ways of doing things. "If you are committed to some kind of risk, like this Dogme, then you are starting on a new level every time. It is meant not as a law for everyone to follow, but as a cure, as an opportunity other people might find inspiration in, so that they might 'undress' and get back to basics. Søren, who is in his fifties, he's done something like fifty-five features, expensive films. He is quite well dressed, so it was quite obvious to ask him to undress. Our fourth brother, Kristian Levring, did his film in English in Namibia, Africa. He lives in London and has been making commercials for a number of years, so he's also very well dressed. The pitiful thing about me," laments Vinterberg, "is that I am not so long out of the Danish Film School, so for me it felt more natural to work within these borders. But there is a problem. It seems that the ideas of Dogme scare people more than they attract them."

"I know this to be true," confirms Levring, "because I have shot a lot of commercials. You can be in Beijing, Moscow, Los Angeles, or Paris—you always end up shooting the same way. Meaning, there is a specific way of lighting, of camera movement, of everything. It's becomes the way to control and predict a page of a script."

So far, true enough. The rest of the Dogme originals include Levring's *The King Is Alive* (Dogme #4), with Jennifer Jason Leigh and Romain Bohringer, and Kragh-Jacobsen's baroque love story *Mifune* (Dogme #3), which won top honors at the 1999 Berlin Film

"**Lars von Trier** has got more sense than to invite me to do a Dogme film. I like those films he does—I particularly liked *The Celebration*—but I do think that these guys are just slightly inventing the wheel. Some of us have been doing these things subtly for quite a while. Yes, to get out there and shoot quickly is great—I made lots of films for television on 16mm—and technology will make its way, but at the end of the day, I like celluloid, the 24 frames a second. I'm not that keen to work digitally. I don't have a problem with the cumbersome industrial process of filmmaking. To me, if you learn how to use it, it's liberating. I don't feel compromised by it and I enjoy assimilating its problems. As long we can go on making films within a disciplined medium, I'll be very happy."

**MIKE LEIGH** / Writer/director, *Topsy Turvy, Naked*

Festival (at the 2001 Berlin Film Festival, the fifth Danish Dogme film, Lone Scherfig's Dogme #12, *Italian for Beginners* also won the Silver Bear). Besides Korine, only one other outsider has undertaken the process, actor Jean-Marc Barr (godfather to von Trier's twin sons, he has appeared in the director's *Europa, Breaking the Waves* and *Dancer in the Dark*). Barr directed the first official French Dogme film, the aptly titled *Lovers* (Dogme #5), starring the gamine Elodie Bouchez (*Dream Life of Angels*).

Barr, 38, who calls Paris home, is prepping his second film, *Too Much Flesh,* to star Rosanna Arquette, in Chicago. Barr says that especially for a greenhorn like him, the relatively low-budget aspect of Dogme was a terrific entree into the major motion picture arena. "Lars and Thomas have given this format credibility," says Barr excitedly. "We wrote our script in a month and a half, financed it in ten days through Canal+ and TF1 International, shot in twenty days, and cut in six weeks, so the whole process took six to seven months which, as you know, is completely unorthodox."

To date there have been twenty-four official Dogme films proudly listed on the Dogme 95 Web site, but the dearth of interest from more established directors is not for lack of effort, says Vinterberg. "Lars sent out invitations on Dogme's behalf, and he's not humble, he sent them to Bergman, big guys like that. When I was at Cannes, I actually asked Scorsese. We spoke a lot about the Dogme concept, so I said, 'Join up. Jump over the barricades.' He laughed, and was drawn away by his bodyguards. End of conversation."

Nor is there a paucity of media awareness. It has drawn fascination and debate, sparking love, hate and relentless international media attention, with articles in *Newsweek, Variety* and *Cahiers du Cinema. Time* magazine quoted Steven Spielberg championing the ethic, enthusing about the possibility of making his own Dogme film. Just imagine *Jurassic Park* with real dinosaurs, filmed in natural light. Most Hollywood players, possibly fearing a cold light on their own concepts, dismiss Dogme as a calculated, publicity-seeking example of "the emperor's new clothes" hucksterism. Admittedly, von Trier knows a thing or two about showmanship. In his twenties, at the Danish Film School, he antagonized his teachers and foreshadowed his future as a provocateur by adopting a false "von" as part of his name, tweaking the feigned grandeur of fellow faux cinema-grandees Erich "von" Stroheim and Josef "von" Sternberg. Cannes 1998 offered a perfect example of Danish irreverence—the Dogme 95 logo.

Literally, "in a pig's eye," its design featured a chubby porcine rear with a huge blinking eye in the anus, and sparked heated discussion and scathing commentary. Some even sniffed condescendingly that the splashy Danes should add commandment #11: Full frontal male nudity is mandatory.

"Well...yes! Why not?" von Trier riposted ingenuously. Walking the walk, talking the talk, the dean of Dogme had himself shown up and stripped down to direct *The Idiots*. "I had no problem being naked," he shrugs. "It was great, very '60s, '70s. By the end everyone was so tired of seeing me naked—'Put on some clothes Lars,' they'd say." He laughs. "But I think it helped them anyway, because some of the nude scenes are quite relaxed." After a well-timed beat, he leans forward and purrs, "They don't have any penetration in *The Celebration*, do they? We had this very famous Danish journalist, female, ask me on television, 'Why is penetration important?' I said, 'You are asking *me*?' She is very well known for..." von Trier, obviously holding a juicy bit of gossip, hesitates, then moves on. "Anyway, I said to her, 'You are asking me why is penetration important?'" His mouth twitches wryly. "'That's a very good question.' It is true, in this regard, I did break the rules. Because, I'm afraid, it's difficult to find actors who are...ah...able, you know, to function in all these aspects, so some of

the 'work' is doubled. It gave me no pleasure, because yeah, that's not very Dogme. I would say that it might go against the intention, but there is not a rule saying that you cannot use a fake prick. Besides, it's kind of a live prick, right?"

Written in four days, shot 80 percent by the director on a hand-held DV camera [a Sony VX 1000], *The Idiots*, he says, is "a film by idiots about idiots for idiots." Von Trier says that he was seeking lost innocence, attempting to capture the lightness and enjoyment of the French New Wave and Beatles-era Swinging London period. The film, however, explores concepts of normalcy and societal codes by focusing on a commune of white middle-class adults who unlock their creative energy and emotional needs by pretending to be retarded, evincing their solidarity, usually in public, by entering into a frenzied, near religious collapse they term "spazzing." I ask how he got his actors to go the distance. Von Trier playfully counters my query by offering to let me experience one of his directorial secrets—hypnosis. It's a control technique he says he used with some actors early on. "The American approach would be the power you have over another human being, but this is a normal technique. It's not a big deal, it's kind of European...and probably more effective," he adds teasingly, "with an accent like mine." He numbers German filmmaker

Werner Herzog [*Hearts of Glass,* who also plays the father in Korine's *julien donkey-boy*], among practitioners of the art, as well as director Bille August's father, whom, he points out, was a traveling hypnotist with the circus. Perhaps most significant for von Trier is that fellow filmmaker and Dane Carl Dreyer employed the technique on stage actress Maria Falconetti [who found working with Dreyer to be such an intense experience, she never made another film], the Joan of his silent classic, *The Passion of Joan of Arc,* the director's inspiration for his own *Breaking the Waves.* "Of course, to get that look," von Trier footnotes, "Dreyer also had her

have sex before shooting. The hypnotism itself is not so strange. The difficult part is being the one who is hypnotized."

In this regard, he confesses, the Dogme rules are custom made for him. "All these rules are designed for me to give away control," says von Trier, who by dint of word and action has become notorious for his Woody Allenish anxieties and phobias. "Technically, it's always been very important to me how the colors of the film look. It's a great relief to have a rule saying: 'It's color film, you can't do anything about it.' If you see all the rules, they are more or less designed for me not to do what I have been doing for a long time."

All agree that this new concentration shifted onto the actors often necessitates extensive use of improvisation, which focuses on the emotional force of the acting. Factor in the handheld camera and the visual results are often grainy images, chaotic camera movements, a bombardment of unstable set-ups, energetic jump-cutting and frequently visible sound equipment. This combination gives the films a raw, pseudo-documentary feel, but is that what the public wants to see? And does that even matter? The

"Because of that support, we allow ourselves to make films without wor-

implication is that such a rarified form of filmmaking emerged because Denmark's government generously supports the arts, not only as an economic incentive, but as support for the national culture.

rying so much about audiences and ratings and such," says Søren Kragh-Jacobsen, slightly distracted by the attention of passing well-wishers attending the Edinburgh Film Festival where his *Mifune* has been screening. We're comparing notes over coffee, after colliding in the artificial twilight of the Edinburgh Sheraton's bar. He looks over my shoulder as he speaks, his gaze lingering on new director Tim Roth, who is energetically sharing his views on cinematic excellence with his current listener, as his film *The War Zone* [written by Alexander Stuart] is also showing at the festival this year. "Dogme," he begins again, breaking away away from Roth, returning to topic at hand, "is not a style—it's a set of inspiring rules. Before Dogme, I swore I would never make another picture again. I can't speak for anyone else, but for me, it has changed everything."

Back in Copenhagen, I wonder if von Trier worries that people will lose interest in Dogme 95, especially as his *Dancer in the Dark*, his post-Dogme musical, has been released in America before the earlier, censorship-plagued *The Idiots*. "Maybe they will like *Dancer* better," he retorts quickly. "There's a lot of singing, dancing. Lots of bloodshed. And it all takes place in America in 1964. Maybe it will be better for my career than *The Idiots*. I saw this Dogme cartoon in a New York paper which equates it with making primitive, cheap art. That's terrible. What's more terrible," he finishes tartly, "is that they keep referring to us as the four 'Dogme Brothers.' It makes us sound like a barbershop quartet." He shakes his head, snapping his fingers in syncopated time as he begins to sing. "Dooo...dooo...wah...be my life's companion and you will never grow old.... Okay, that's enough of that," he says briskly, grabbing his jacket and hustling me out the door. "This is boring. *Very* boring. No more singing. No more Dogme. I have work to do."

> If the doctrine appears to be different things to all people, says Jesper Jargil, whose documentary *The Humiliated* follows the making of *The Idiots*, that's because it is. Jargil is currently editing another feature, *The Exhibited,* a behind-the-scenes view of all three completed Dogme films. "For Lars, it was almost like a religion," he says. "For Thomas, it was to have fun. For Søren it was a personal test. You asked if, in Denmark, we get a little tired of hearing about all this. Sure we do. When you think about these rules, some of them are really clever, some are just irritating. I personally think the one about filming and recording the sound at the same time makes everything too difficult."

Jargil, who helped cast *The Idiots* and was cameraman for part of its shoot, recalls one particular episode. "Sometimes, to make things more practical, the production team had to 'arrange' things a bit. Not the big issues. But if Lars finds out, on even the little ones, that something has been played with, he cannot live with that. We were out on location, and the crew got back before Lars and the actors. They knew they were going to shoot the scene up in this attic, and they knew the light was going to fade before the actors arrived, but luckily up in the attic they found a lamp.

"Great," says Jargil. "We say, we found this on location (as the rules dictate). This is *really* a Dogme lamp. But there was no place to plug it in, the cord was not long enough, and there was no extension cord in the house. The soundman says he's got a cord down in the sound car, and we tell him to go get it. So he gets this huge cord, we plug it in somewhere and run it upstairs. Then Lars comes and sees this and says 'What is this cord?' The soundman goes deep red. And Lars gets angry, really angry. When the actors arrive he tells them we need some light up there and sends them over to the neighbor's house to borrow a cord. It took half an hour for them to get that and when they brought it back, Lars made a long speech about what is a Dogme extension cord and what is not. Acting-wise, I think it was a fantastic experience. But for their personal lives, I think it was a terrible period, because nobody had ever tried to work that way. A director can be sort of a dictator, and you have to follow. And Lars has a very strong personality."

Peter Aalbaek Jensen, with Vibeke Vinderlov, is von Trier's long time producer and friend. A tall, normally expansive, robust gentle-man, usually encountered with a fat cigar lodged between his teeth, Jensen looks uncommonly fatigued today sitting outside Zentropa's main offices. "No, I'm fine," he protests, laughing and wrapping me in a huge bear hug, though we've met but once before. "I'm just tired, because I'm not drinking." And because, he discreetly fails to mention, he has just endured a huge public battle with von Trier for going behind the direc-tor's back and color correcting the print of *The Idiots,* which has since been restored by the rigorous von Trier to its pristine, Dogme state.

"How could I do it?" he asks. "For the sake of money. It was not possible to see the goddamn actors. I was doing him a favor, but," adds Jensen, pushing his glasses firmly in place, "he was extremely pissed. That is the distasteful conflict between art and money." An avowed philistine, Jensen is far more comfortable dealing with the latter. Although he claims he is still befuddled by all the fuss, he has rightly sensed that there is money to be made and has therefore taken it upon himself to develop the commercial side of the ideology.

> Toward this end is Zentropa's porno arm, Puzzy Power. "It's my idea," Jensen boasts, "but Lars thinks it would be fun to do a porno movie, Dogme-style. And in the UK we made an agreement with a company called Wave to work with the Dogme ideal. Why not? To me, the most important things that have happened in film are *The Blair Witch Project* in America [reputed to have earned creators Ed Sanchez and Daniel Myrick mondo mega-buck status], and Dogme. It's part of the same consciousness, you could say."

What Jensen has rightly concluded is that with the rapid advancements in digital video technology, plus the arrival of desktop editing systems, and the inevitable transition of television to digital broadcasting, the digital revolution has begun, ready to provide more visual bang for your buck, pound or yen.

> Because Dogme 95 forbids all forms of Hollywood studio trickery, the result is a gloss-free, pseudo-documentary feeling that dovetails nicely with the growing demand for reality-type programming. This voyeuristic "Big Brother" aesthetic will not fade away anytime soon. Its digital antecedents are in the big screen films of gearheads Spielberg and Lucas, and (non-Dogme) DV releases including the aforementioned, box-office busting *Blair Witch Project,* plus UK directors Mike Figgis' *TimeCode* and the handheld ethos of Michael Winterbottom's celluloid adventure *Wonderland.*

Whereas previously one could be overwhelmed by the financial, physically weighty demands of a traditional 35mm camera and crew, an impulsive filmmaker can now tote a tiny digicam and capture the blissful "non-actory" moments of a human being with no idea that he or she is being taped. Privacy issues notwithstanding, Harmony Korine took this possibility to the next creative level by utilizing a special PAL package comprised of nine different cameras, created especially for his cinematographer Anthony Dod Mantle, with features including night-vision and a special spy camera mounted in a pair of eyeglasses.

## "I think until *The Idiots*, [Godard] thought what I was doing was RUBBISH. Now, maybe, I've kind of...well, come home"

Says Jensen, "It has made the making of films more of a democratic event. Yes, people say 'cheap filmmaking,' but if you want to, you can still make really expensive movies with the Dogme. For me, for a silly little country that makes silly little movies, to have this big noise spread around the world is a whole lot of fun." Dogme, Jensen adds, has certainly enabled von Trier to be more fluid in his visual approach. "On *Dancer* Robby Mueller [also cinematographer for *Breaking the Waves*] handled the lighting, but Lars was the camera operator. The handheld camera rule from Dogme made it possible for him to have more contact with the actors, instead of just looking at the monitor and screaming at them. Things used to go from the storyboard directly to the camera, which was good to look at, but boring. With this, there is nothing but the actors, their talent, the director and the story. Nobody can hide behind anything, and there are no excuses. Sure, it makes him more vulnerable, but it's also given him a lot of freedom to create. And the actors love it."

As the theory goes, the strength of American filmmaking comes from the fact that it is an industry. The cachet of European filmmaking is derived from its individualism. When it tries to compete on Hollywood terms, it becomes Euro-pudding. [Or *Notting Hill.*] The Dogme manifesto underscores this quandary by pointing out that the French anti-bour-geois New Wave of the 1960s eventually mainstreamed because its foundations were based on the bourgeois perception of art. Could the arrogance of Dogme 95 become bourgeois? Vinterberg has stated that he would be proud if it did, because it would mean that it had been 'big' first. "It's a natural evolution from avant-garde to mainstream," he explains. "There's a reaction, [the reaction] becomes convention, and everyone falls asleep."

In fact, says von Trier, Godard himself asked for and screened *The Idiots.* "I think until *The Idiots*, [Godard] thought what I was doing was rubbish. Now, maybe, I've kind of...well, come home," he remarks, obviously pleased. "The New Wave is a wave that's always coming. They didn't put anything down on a piece of paper. We are doing it a little bit more Dogmatic, in a sense." Von Trier says he has no plans to do another Dogme film (although he agrees with Jensen that it would be especially interesting to do a porno film with that discipline). Do one, he says, and if you learn from your experience, according to all adherents, there is no need to do another. It's always possible to renew the vows if creative bloating occurs. There is no cover or minimum attached to Dogme's Pritikin-strict canon.

"People ask, 'Is Dogme tongue in cheek?'" continues von Trier. "Yes, it is an experiment, but I can only tell you, I take it very seriously. [To me] it's like horseback riding; here in Denmark we have a discipline called 'school riding' [a formal English equestrian training]. For people who are interested in horses this is very interesting. I'm sure that the experience of this strange way of riding can be used otherwise in life. So, [like Dogme] if you want to do it, you should follow the rules, or else it is nonsense. If you get carried away and ride over the prairie, be my guest. I think there's a certain beauty to that. I don't think there's any point in merely provoking. Any kind of discussion, any thinking about the media and how you're working with it is a good thing, and that is what can provoke. It did in Cannes—everybody was talking about it. You may think it's worthless, but here you are, you're still arguing about *why* it's worthless."

One man who certainly isn't quibbling is Korine. For all the ruckus his *julien donkey-boy* caused, Korine says that above all it facilitated an atmosphere within which he could motivate the actors to do their best, to push themselves beyond their limits. A place, he says, lighting up his umpteenth cigarette, that he visits every day. At the intense center of the Dogme-imposed environment, Korine felt secure and safe. "It was really small and intimate, and we were shooting at my grandma's house in a family environment. My Grandma Joyce [who plays Julien's grandmother] enjoyed it even though I'm not sure she knew what the hell was going on or even what a movie is. She was just happy to have people around to cook for and to talk to." They knew the meal was ready, Korine recalls, when their attention was diverted by black smoke and fire issuing from the oven.

With Dogme, it's all part of the movie.

# 10 INSIDER TIPS TO DOGME 95:
## NARRATIVE DIALOGUE LOGISTICS

1. **Make extensive use of improvisation even if it embarrasses your actors.**

   It will flatter the cast, as the film focuses almost entirely on the emotional force of the performers. And it helps you out, especially if it's your first film, as it gets them to work longer hours for the same money. In interviews they will thank you for allowing them to be involved in the process (although they will continue to slag you off to their friends). You get to take credit as a writer for all that brilliant extra dialogue, and you have more material with which to blackmail your actors if need be. If you've hired on famous actors, this will be especially useful for your next non-Dogme feature.

2. **Let someone else hand-hold your camera.**

   Usage of these smaller handheld cameras is a reaction against stuffy, glossy, studio shot features, and the physically restrictive weight of the filmmaking machinery. Read up on your Nouvelle Vague. Remind everyone that the intrusive intimacy of the herky-jerky image and those chaotic movements are inventing new language of cinema…besides, all that "I am the camera" stuff brings you closer to the actors. But, even though those cameras are small they can get damn heavy, especially when you can't afford a tripod. Hiring a DP who is in good physical condition is a very sound idea.

3. **Make sure the color images are grainy.**

   Frequently accompany them with a bombardment of unstable set-ups. The raw visual aesthetic and the lack of *mise en scene* gets you even closer to that imitation of reality. It also adds a sheen of dark drama even to the lightest comedic moments. No one has to know you couldn't afford a lighting package. In post-production it will drive your editor and your transfer house near to madness. During this approximately twelve week period, supplying them with vast quantities of their secret vice is a good idea.

### 4. Edit to show the flaws.

Energetic jump-cutting and frequently visible sound equipment combine to give the films a raw, pseudo-documentary feel. This way your post-production facility and your editor can't blame themselves for hating you; optical work and filters were not in your budget anyway. Later on, spiritedly insist that the resultant aesthetic was clearly the intention, as it acted as a subtextual emotion, an additional character if you will, within the nonlinear framework of the story.

### 5. Reference the Nouvelle Vague and John Cassavetes.

No one who has a life other than the cinema has seen all the films from the French New Wave, or completely understands the reasons behind or can even pronounce, *Cahiers du Cinema*. But they've seen photos and think that Belmondo is very cool and sexy. Most haven't seen Cassavetes' film work and most can't spell his last name either, but they've seen photos and also sense him to be very cool and sexy. Throwing in a silent film director such as F.W. Murnau will also act as a confusing, ironic counterpoint.

### 6. If you must shoot on location, do it in a foreign country.

That way you'll get to travel a little bit after the production wraps. And your creditors won't be able to reach you as easily. Do not give them the number of your tri-band mobile.

### 7. Name drop other Dogme auteurs and their DV choices.

Casually. Like, "When Lars and I spoke over coffee last week about his Sony VX1000 and his transfer to Academy 35mm at Denmark's Hokus Bogus," or, "Before I tell you his joke about color timing at Swiss Effects, let me tell you Harmony's hilarious story about when he first picked up a Sony PD100...."

### 8. Confess to a non-generic fatal flaw.

Being too handsome or too smart has a nasty boomerang effect—we all know that all too well don't we? Scrape up something original. And don't even think about saying you won't fly in a plane, ever. That one is von Trier's and he'll get really irritated if you try to bogart his phobia. Try to sound vulnerable, damaged and humble, even though you really don't mean it. The world likes their genius heroes to be deeply flawed; it makes their tumble from grace even more exciting. Paranoia and cruelty due to a corrosive relationship with your mother only works if your film is good, so be careful.

## 9. Tell everyone you run into that it's your movie.

Mine, mine, mine! Even though the Dogme rules forbid a director to be credited on screen, there's no rule that says you can't print it on t-shirts, or talk about how the lack of credit thing works in every interview you do. They did it; so can you. Confuse people further by saying your next film will be a celluloid story and you're going to shoot with the biggest, most cumbersome cameras you can find.

## 10. Make sure people know that taking on Dogme 95's Vow of Chastity doesn't mean you can't date.

That particular heading in the Dogme canon often confuses admirers at film festivals who want to show their deep, deep admiration for the risks you've taken with your work. Remind them Dogme is a form of "stripped down" filmmaking and they'll probably get the hint. (What's all that cinematic purity for if you can't have a little Babylonian fun with it afterwards?)

# ORIGINAL DOGME

## HARMONY KORINE

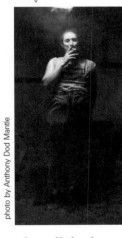

photo by Anthony Dod Mantle

"I make my films from the inside out," drawls Harmony Korine, Manhattan's favorite bad-boy auteur in a slow, gravelly voice that Kerouac might have coveted. "I have to in order to blur the line between what really happened and what is made up, manipulated, fictitious, and completely correct, until I don't recognize it anymore."

Slight of build and disarmingly fresh-faced, Korine's notoriety ignited at age eighteen when he had a chance encounter with photographer Larry Clark in Manhattan's Washington Square Park. Though he'd only completed a semester at NYU, Korine dropped out to write the script for Clark's 1995 film *Kids,* a provocative portrait of sexually active teenagers. Two years later Korine assumed the auteur mantle with his own *Gummo,* a hypnotically scuzzy journey of two glue-sniffing kids who sell dead cats, which immediately established him as an anarchic lightning rod in the filmmaking community.

Korine extended the discomfort zone with *julien donkey-boy*, another intimate, darkly skewed tale, which Korine shot under the auspices of Dogme 95. Based in part on the life of his uncle, an institutionalized schizophrenic, *julien* focuses on the inner life of a mentally disturbed man who finds salvation working in a school for the blind. Lensed primarily in Korine's grandmother's house in Queens by cinematographer Anthony Dod Mantle, the film revels in a variety of low-tech imagery (obtained with up to thirty different kinds of video cameras, including a variety of nifty "spy" devices) and a nonlinear storytelling technique that is both infuriating and lyrically arresting. It was also largely improvised by a cast that includes *Trainspotting*'s Ewen Bremner in the title role, longtime collaborator Chloë Sevigny as his sweetly dreamy pregnant sister, Korine's grandmother Joyce as Julien's grandmother, and icon/filmmaker Werner Herzog in an funny/scary turn as Julien's abusive father.

Bremner proved a brilliant choice for the titular hero, and prepared for the role by visiting Korine's uncle at New York's Creedmoor Psychiatric Center and working in a hospital for six weeks. But Bremner was not the director's first choice. "I was going to try and get my uncle out of the institution for the movie, but that proved impossible," says Korine. "I was nervous about using Ewen because he has this thick Scottish accent, and is certainly not schizophrenic…it got really scary toward the end," relates Korine. "I wouldn't have liked it if he was the kind of actor that switches on and off, but he was in character all through the shooting and towards the end I was nervous that he had gone…off. I saw no trace of Ewen, and I wanted him back. I was glad when the movie was finished."

> Even if it's chaos, there has to be a way to ANTICIPATE the chaos, to reorganize it, and then make SENSE of it.

Utilizing the rapid-paced approach Dogme provides took the actors to a place they wouldn't have been able to reach otherwise. There was a screenplay, Korine says, but one far different than the norm. "There were very detailed scene descriptions, describing what should/could happen, so the story could evolve and the narrative progress. But other than that, it was really up to the actors. We shot for hours using video, which sounds chaotic," he adds, exhaling a long plume of cigarette smoke which forms a penumbra over his head, "but, there has to be a certain system for me. Even if it's chaos, there has to be a way to anticipate the chaos, to reorganize it, and then make sense of it. People always speak of 'truth in cinema,' but that's a fallacy. It's all subjective. The truth is, if I didn't have film, I'd be a lost soul."

**Pessimists worry that the digitalization of the medium spells the end of movies. Utopians prophesy their ultimate democratization. What do you think?**

I do not care one bit. Technology bores me. It's just more films of the same kind...don't let any of it fool you. It is only a machine. It steals from man what it can never give back. I will just react and or hibernate.

**Will celluloid go the way of vinyl?**

I hope so. the answers are in the crackles and the scratch- es. Like i have said for years now, i am a "mistakist" artist. All the best artists of this era are. "Mistakism" is the greatest form of all. Post-modernism has long been adopted and dwarfed by "mistakism" but i have been saying this since I was 18, I am bored by it all. When I am dead perhaps people will latch on.

**Do you see cinema today as an art form?**

I don't see cinema today.

**You have created intense tapestries of sound and image, yet that's not necessarily the story. What are the themes that call to you? What moves you? What do you find daunting?**

I have no insight to share. It is all in my work. I find everything else daunting. I am not exaggerating. I wish i was born a happier person; I wish i could have been born Meg Ryan. I want to be her. She is so happy and this makes me envy her every second of every day. Harmony Korine is worshipping at the altar of "When Harry Met Sally."

Werner Herzog in julien donkey-boy.
photo by Anthony Dod Mantle

**Is the feeling of authenticity, a current concern in cinema and the holy grail of the *cinéma vérité* movement, a product of techniques and rules as rigorous as the choreography of an MGM musical or the editing of a Hitchcock thriller?**

This question would be better asked of a Chinese person.

**There have been many good movies recently. Do you think this signals a return to the heyday of '70s filmmaking?**

No. To hell with '70s cinema idolatry and to hell with each and every one of your heydays.

**Do you believe that filmmaking must be linked to
a certain kind of truth, or a certain kind of risk?**

Yes.

**Relative to Dogme 95, what do you think
of *Dancer in the Dark*? Can you see the
post-Dogme transformation in von Trier's work
and in yours?**

This question would be better asked of a Northern Korean
censor...but Lars is a special man. I take my hat off to any
provocateur who has in equal measure talent. Why and how
should i answer this question? Yes i can. I still love the brothers of Dogme 95.

**You've said you enjoy using improvisation in
your work. Have you ever longed to work within
an ultra-strict framework?**

Yes.

**Have you ever lifted a scene from someone?**

I am not yet strong enough to lift an entire scene. I have lifted several half scenes and one three-quarter scene, but
one day I will lift an entire one. You must remember, even
though I am a man, I am still very slight and small boned. To lift
an entire scene requires long hours of focus and training and
I get bored very quickly.

**What do you think about current DV films from
other filmmakers, e.g.: Mike Figgis' *TimeCode*,
Miguel Arteta's *Chuck & Buck*, et. al?**

I told you I don't care. If what "they" do is direct films, I am
of another trade. Not just these men you have mentioned...
although I have nothing in particular against them. In fact i
have never even heard of them. I hope you understand this,
and do not take it in the fashion of Yves Saint-Laurent.

**The word "genre" has become the most abused
word in cinema language. How can that change?**

I don't care about these questions. I just want people to
realize that I simply do the things I do because no else
does. Because real life is a disappointment to me, it always
has been constant misery and suffering, and not worth living
if it weren't for God allowing me to write and direct as I
please. Other than that, I do not care to pontificate or rep-

resent some kind of false restless spirit that has led to a new "Nouvelle Vague" of even more bullshit...and I am certainly no spokesman for that or anything else.

**Historically, what is your favorite period of filmmaking? Favorite filmmakers? Actors?**

When Mao died. Carl Dreyer and Buster Keaton. Alain Delon and Zeppo Marx.

**Much like the "New Wave," do you think that this interest in the DV aesthetic is emerging for a particular cultural or political reason?**

I don't care.

**Whom do you find inspirational? In film, or any walk of life.**

The Red Army Faction. The Bader-Mienhoff gang. I am writing a book on Steppin' Fetchit (the first black actor who starred alongside Will Rodgers), the name of my novel will be called, "Steppin Fetchit: A Man Named After A Race Horse."

**After your experience making *julien donkey-boy*, how do you feel about more traditional forms of filmmaking?**

JDB was a very traditional film, isn't that obvious? It was the complete directory of the "mistakist" tradition.

**As a culture, is our appetite for reality matched only by our craving for fantasy?**

Please, I feel like I am losing a bit more life with every question asked.

**When someone's lifework is the creation of 'fantasy,' what happens to cinema? How does it affect the audience? Does it induce us to forget the difference between seeing and dreaming?**

Jesus, I have a razor to my wrist at this very moment.

**Walter Benjamin said that the best way to discover a city is to get intelligently lost in it. Do you feel that is the best way to approach filmmaking?**

He also said, "The greatest novel of the century would consist entirely of other peoples' quotations." I like that one better. Benjamin was actually my mother's second cousin. In one of his letters to my dead grandmother Elaine, from Prague, shortly after he completed his *Arcades* project, he wrote that he wanted to finish out his years as a boy scout leader in the name of a Zionist militia. When he killed himself, inside his wallet my grandmother's brother Jakob found only a picture of his mother and a twelve-year-old boy fondling his testicles in a strawberry patch.

**Do you feel that filmmaking is viewed as a romantic profession?**

Because romance is so profound, ask God yourself, only he knows the answers you are looking for and he is probably on pins and needles waiting to answer them for you.

**What is your next challenge?**

Isn't it obvious. Must I really explain any further...? (love always, harmony Korine)

## SØREN KRAGH-JACOBSEN >>>

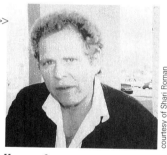

courtesy of Shari Roman

Søren Kragh-Jacobsen's *Mifune* garnered accolades worldwide, including three European Film Awards and the Silver Bear at the Berlin Film Festival in 1999. But *Mifune* was a success story that almost never happened. Just prior to shooting the film, Kragh-Jacobsen was in a state of complete film hate.

A seasoned feature director and writer (as well as a former Danish pop star), Kragh-Jacobsen made his debut in 1978 with *Do You Wanna See My Beautiful Navel*, followed by a succession of other features, including *The Island on Bird Street*. The making of *Bird Street*, however, was such a strangling experience that the 53-year-old director swore that he would never make another film. *Ever*. The oath was quickly forgotten when he was drawn into making his award-winning film *Mifune* under Dogme 95.

Written in two months with young Danish writer/director Anders Thomas Jensen, the darkly comic tale kicks off when yuppie newlywed Kresten (Anders W. Berthelsen) learns of the death of his father. Leaving his upscale new bride (Sofie Grabol), he returns to his rundown family farm to care for his retarded brother Rud (Jesper Asholt), whom he has convinced years earlier that the great Japanese actor Toshiro Mifune lives in the basement of their home.

Paralleling Akira Kurosawa's *The Seven Samurai*, wherein Mifune plays a bogus Samurai of peasant origins, Kresten attempts to hide his hayseed background from his fashionable new friends. To solve his problem, he engages the housekeeping services of the attractive Liva (Iben Hjejle), a classy hooker on the run from a mysterious stalker. Needless to say, things quickly spiral out of his control.

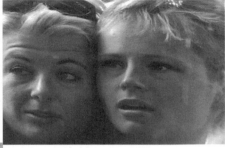

As Kragh-Jacobsen tells it, *Mifune* became the answer to finding his warrior spirit. "I had become so tired of it all," remembers the director. *"Bird Street* was a huge co-production; it was shot in Poland with English, American and German producers. Smell trouble? Making this film was like going on a cure. Now, after *Mifune,* I can't wait to do another film. Limitations create movement, make you stronger," asserts Kragh-Jacobsen. "As I am the oldest of the 'brothers,' the limitations did frustrate me a bit," he admits, "but it was also a relief to work at greater speed, without the burden of a lot of equipment. It encouraged an immediacy and creative freedom."

Although the story was pretty much in place when production began, the actual shooting was far more unpredictable. "If we didn't have available light indoors, we moved the scene out into the garden," he recounts. "One morning we shot in a turnip field, while behind the camera my friend played the accordion as all these cars raced by us. It was wonderful! Filmmaking must always be linked to a certain degree of risk."

*>> The women of Mifune.*
*photos by Anthony Dod Mantle*

Indeed, with *Mifune,* Kragh-Jacobsen didn't emulate his Dogme buddies by shooting in DV. Instead, he shot on 35mm, and the film's visual style is rich and carefully paced. The credit goes to DP Anthony Dod Mantle, whose cinematography on several Dogme films has rendered him a spokesman for the Dogme aesthetic. With *Mifune,* however, both Kragh-Jacobsen and Mantle opted for a sense of grace not evident in the restless style of the film's antecedents.

"'You can't shoot on film' was never one of the rules," protests Kragh-Jacobsen emphatically. "Yes, DV is easier to work with. You can be more agile, and use fewer set-up shots. Yes, you do have to approach everything differently when you are working with a single, very heavy, 35mm camera. But really, it was Thomas and Lars who first broke the rules by not doing their projects on film." Kragh-Jacobsen explains that this is because digital video engenders a certain aesthetic, which in the transfer to film forces a certain visual "tampering" that violates the Dogme ethos. Point of order, anyone?

The important distinction in Kragh-Jacobsen's mind was that *Mifune* was always a celluloid story, and that fact took precedence over the tendency shared by his fellow DV devotees. "We are four different directors," he shrugs, "who have made four different films. Maybe I made the softer movie. Maybe it's a bit old-fashioned, but so what? I'm not so keen on these small cameras.... You can't see everything in the frame and you can't really follow the story as well."

He adds glibly, "Of course, Americans love DV because it looks so arty."

*"One morning we shot in a turnip field, while behind the camera my friend played the ACCORDION as all these cars raced by us. It was wonderful! Filmmaking must always be LINKED to a certain degree of risk."*

As for von Trier, who counters that Kragh-Jacobsen is the one who "broke the rules" since he was initially the chief advocate of the low-budget flexibility of DV filming, Kragh-Jacobsen retorts quickly, "Lars is lying." He pauses, "It's so weird, so typical, Lars saying something like that. I love him, but it's Lars who likes working digitally. Sure, we did break some of the rules in *Mifune*, like kicking some chickens across the yard to get them in the shot, but shooting in 35mm is not one of the rules we broke."

Given the international controversy over the Dogme rules, some critics wonder if it's just a commercial gimmick. Kragh-Jacobsen demurs, stressing that the doctrine was born out of the harsh self-analysis of its founders regarding their culpability in cinematic mediocrity. "You can say the whole Dogme concept is a game," muses Kragh-Jacobsen, "but it's not funny, cheating on this game. It is all meant as a way to bring you closer to creativity and spontaneity in your work. What's the point in cheating yourself of that? Dogme, for me, has done what it is supposed to do. I love making movies again."

### How do you understand Dogme-style film-making?

Dogme is not a style, it's a set of inspiring rules which have many colors. Originally, there were four Danish directors who formed this group; Thomas Vinterberg, who made *Festen*; Lars von Trier, who made *The Idiots*; Kristian Levring, who has made *The King Is Alive*; and myself.

### *Festen* and *The Idiots* were shot on digital video and then transferred to 35mm. Is that a Dogme rule?

No, it's just easier. You can shoot more, and it's a bit more free in certain regards.

### Why is the film called *Mifune*?

I found the house where we filmed the movie on the day Toshiro Mifune died. I wanted to give the old master one last part and put him in my film. He really entertained me over the years.

### With Dogme 95 attracting so much attention, Danish film seems to be on an upsurge.

It's been good for the actors too.

Hollywood has been snapping up a lot of our actors. Iben, who plays the housekeeper in my film, was in the Stephen Frears' film *High Fidelity* with John Cusack.

Maybe it's because we do have a lot of film subsidies, and we don't make expensive films. Also, the state sees the support as support for the culture. So we allow ourselves to make films without worrying so much about audiences and ratings. And that's really good, because out of that comes a Lars von Trier.

### Would you change anything in *Mifune*?

Yes and no. I've made something like ten films and I don't always love them when they're finished, but when they are finished they have a new life. Their own life. There are always mistakes, but I wouldn't change anything about the way I did this film. For me, it was like being in film school again. But I won't make another Dogme film. After you make one, you don't make another one. It has done what it is supposed to do. You can bring some of your experiences to the next one. Ah, but who knows? Who can tell?

# THE CONFESSION OF SØREN KRAGH-JACOBSEN

As one of the DOGME 95 brethren and co-signatory of the Vow of Chastity I feel moved to confess to the following transgressions of the aforesaid Vow during the production of Dogme #3, *Mifune*. Please note that the film has been approved as a Dogme work, as only one genuine breach of the rules has actually taken place. The rest may be regarded as moral breaches.

I confess to having made one take with a black drape covering a window. This is not only the addition of a property, but must also be regarded as a kind of lighting arrangement.

I confess to moving furniture and fittings around the house.

I confess to having taken with me a number of albums of my favourite cartoon series as a youth, *Linda & Valentin*.

I confess to helping to chase the neighbour's free-range hens across our location and including them in the film.

I confess that I brought a photographic image from an old lady from the area and hung it in a prominent position in one scene: not as part of the plot, but more as a selfish, spontaneous, pleasurable whim.

I confess to borrowing a hydraulic platform from a painter, which we used for the only two bird's-eye overview shots in the film.

I do solemnly declare that in my presence the remainder of Dogme #3, *Mifune* was produced in accordance with the Vow of Chastity.

I also point out that the film has been approved by DOGME 95 as a Dogme film, as in real terms no more than a single breach of the rules has been commited. The rest may be regarded as moral transgressions.

Copenhagen, 20 January 1999
Søren Kragh-Jacobsen

"**The Dogme** approach helped me refine my own voice after a number of years with less personal work and gave me the euphoric feeling of playing with the film medium, in the way I have always admired the Italians for being so good at. ❖ I began by specifically writing the script for five actors with whom I had worked with very closely; I knew they had a talent for improvisation, which was especially needed as some scenes in the script were not altogether finished. Many incidents and back stories in the script were inspired by actual events or are autobiographical elements, which slowly became formed by adherence to the Dogme rules. Whenever things changed—the weather, the mood, the feeling for a character—I would change the scene instead of trying to solve the problem. The interesting thing about *Italian for Beginners* is, although the Dogme rules were very important in the way in which I created the film, visually, it ended up looking like fairly normal production."

**LONE SCHERFIG** / Writer/Director, Dogme #12, *Italian for Beginners*

## JEAN-MARC BARR

Born in Germany in 1960, the son of an American Air Force soldier and a French mother, Jean-Marc Barr was captain of his high school football team and "did the whole American thing," living in the States for twenty years before heading off to Europe to study at the Guild School of Drama in London. Appearing first in small roles in Bruce Beresford's *King David* and John Boorman's *Hope and Glory,* his breakout role came in 1988, as the young diver in Luc Besson's *The Big Blue.* His collaborations with Lars von Trier, as lead in 1991's *Europa* [American title, *Zentropa*], followed by ensemble roles in the *Breaking the Waves* and *Dancer in the Dark* introduced his face to a wider audience. Residing originally in the U.S., then in London, and now in Paris, Barr has begun directing, and made his debut behind the camera in 1999 with *Lovers,* which he shot under the restrictions of the Dogme manifesto. Filmed in Paris and now classified as Dogme #5, *Lovers* focuses on a young French girl, played by Elodie Bouchez (*The Dream Life of Angels*), and a Yugoslavian immigrant, portrayed by Sergej Trifunovic, who fall in love despite their cultural differences.

**How did you end up directing a Dogme film?**

As an actor I had become very passive. Did my job. I was getting quite bored with it. Success is great, but if you're an actor, you're not going to get very far by just doing pictures where you're killing monsters and beating up people. It's better to take risks. I was influenced by Godard and these other directors taking chances. After *The Big Blue* people wondered why I didn't do bigger pictures. Instead of going to Hollywood, I did *Orpheus Descending* with Vanessa Redgrave in the West End. It was directed by Peter Hall, and it also brought me to Lars, which brought me to the anti-aesthetic of *Europa*, which of course brought me to be influenced by Lars. I am godparent to his little sons. Although I don't see him on a regular basis, his dialogue in the cinema— what he believes in—is what Pascal [Arnold], my collaborator, and I believe in, too.

**And then you went to Cannes...**

When Pascal and I saw *The Idiots* and *The Celebration* there, when we saw what could be achieved, we decided it was time to make a picture, that it was a viable opportunity for new filmmakers like ourselves. I love Billy Wilder, Ernst Lubistch; I've always wanted to take that kind of sensibility and transfer it to something modern. All of a sudden, with Lars and Thomas bringing out Dogme, this new approach gained credibility and we got our film financed. Lars knows that cinema is telling a story and trying to touch people, but also that a lot of it is a reaction to technology. He told a beautiful story with good actors and a camera on his shoulder, with good technicians behind him. He let himself go and inspired a whole lot of people. That kind of daring is what keeps me in Europe. You can work with Harmony Korine or Larry Clark, but honestly, there aren't many filmmakers like them in America.

**What was the filmmaking process like for you?**

I thought it would be easier since I come from an acting background, but the first time I held the camera, I was shaking! We had a lot of freedom, but that gave us a lot of responsibility. We discovered that, for the first time in our careers, because the budget was so low and we didn't have a

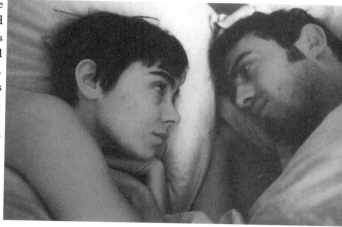

company telling us what to do, we could do whatever we wanted. No restrictions except for the ones we planned on ourselves. Our big challenge was to make a film, to make it economically viable, and do something completely fresh at the same time. We thought an "international" film, rather than a French film, would be the best idea—especially as it was a love story that took place in Paris between a Yugoslavian man who doesn't speak French but speaks English, and a woman who speaks both French and English. Eventually they'd have to communicate in "the world language" of English, which would give it a better chance in the marketplace.

*Elodie Bouchez and Sergei Trifunovic in* Lovers.
courtesy of Jean Marc Barr/Toloda

**You wrote the script in a month and a half?**

That's right. And we financed it in ten days through Canal+ and TF1 for $500,000 [£344,000]. We shot it over three weeks in December. We were able to shoot in the streets of Paris and didn't need extras, because with that little camera and a guy with a boom and the sound people we just blended in with the crowd. The whole process took around seven months, which is completely unorthodox. When we went to Cannes with the film, we sold it to twenty countries and made back our money with the pre-sales to fourteen countries. Pascal and I felt like we were probably getting close to what Mack Sennett was feeling in the 1920s. [Mack Sennett Studios produced such a tremendous volume of slapstick shorts for the likes of Charlie Chaplin, The Keystone Kops, etc., that Sennett earned the moniker, "America's King of Comedy."] This new digital technology was the reason for this freedom. So we decided to do a trilogy on freedom, which is called free-trilogy. The first movie of this trilogy is *Lovers*, which is about freedom to love. The second film, which we shot in America, is called *Too Much Flesh*, which is about freedom of sexuality. And the third part is about freedom of spirit, freedom of thought, which is called *Being Light*.

**Did you break any of the rules in making *Lovers*?**

We got the certification the day before we screened at Cannes! In fact we had to do some changes to make it completely Dogme. *Lovers* had to be seen by the three or four people to get our little diploma. We had to do a letter confession and they'll allow you three or four sins—for example, we thought it was too bourgeois not to put the director's name on it, but in the end we changed it to just the cameraman. The thing that gave us the most trouble was at the end on one of the bridges. We used a portable fluorescent light because it helped us get a better image on the actors' faces.

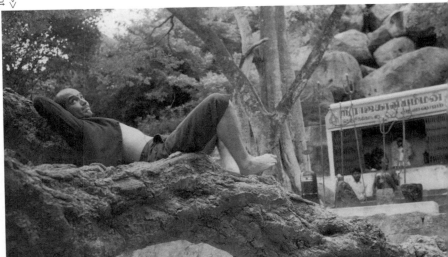

Jean Marc Barr in Being Light
courtesy of Jean Marc Barr/Toloda

## Do you consider Dogme to be a revolutionary approach?

When it came out it, people didn't take it seriously at all. Then people thought it was a marketing gimmick. This is not unusual thinking. I mean, with the advent of the talkies people lost their jobs because their voices weren't up to par, and then they were stunned by the introduction of color film. Dogme is not a revolution. It's more a productive alternative. The filmmakers of the Nouvelle Vague in the '60s were reacting to a cinema that had stunted itself, so the directors took the cameras and produced the films themselves and had complete control. In that sense, Dogme is not a new wave, but it's like a new wave in the sense that technology allows it. In France, we have such a problem because our first-time directors can't get financing. If they want to make a movie they have to go with huge budgets and if they screw up they have to find a new career. Dogme is a great way to make a feature and express yourself creatively without destroying yourself financially. All this with a camera no bigger than a shoebox.

## KRISTIAN LEVRING

"There is so much mystery to Africa," sighs Danish auteur Kristian Levring. "Namibia, where we shot The King Is Alive, is twice as big as France, but there are only 500,000 people, all in the desert." Pining for that great expanse from a small, crowded coffeehouse in London's SoHo district, Levring adds, "There aren't that many places in the world where you can get lost, where the world is still that big."

The King Is Alive is the fourth official addition to the Dogme 95 canon. Shot in story sequence over six weeks in the summer of 1999, the story follows a group of tour bus sightseers (with a cast that includes Jennifer Jason Leigh, Janet McTeer and Bruce Davison) who end up stranded in an abandoned mining town in the middle of nowhere. With faint hope of rescue, the passengers decide to pass the time by staging a play, settling on Shakespeare's gloomy, monolithic King Lear. No barrel of laughs, the play only serves to hurl the panicked collective into chaos as they struggle with emotional and sexual tensions that threaten to push them all to the brink of madness.

"This film is very heavy," admits Levring, who collaborated on the screenplay with *Mifune* scribe Anders Thomas Jensen. "It's about dying, it's about big emotions," he says, adding, "but the amazing thing about the Dogme style is I don't think the actors or myself ever had a more joyful shoot. There are restrictions—there always are when you make a film—but on the other hand there is so much liberty. It's because when you work this way you devote perhaps half an hour to technology, and the other eleven and a half hours to how the scene is evolving and the kind of emotions you're going for." Utilizing three handheld Sony PD 100 miniDV cameras (whose footage he later transferred to 35mm), Levring has seamlessly adhered to the strict tenets of Dogme while lensing some of the most extraordinary and breathtaking imagery ever seen on digital video. Capturing a lush, renaissance-like contrast between inky darkness and the timeless, endlessly shifting architecture of the bleached desert sand, which equally support and mock the fragility of his lost survivors.

Indeed, with his shoulder-length tresses and gentle, bearded face, Levring looks more like an 18th century painter than a 21st century cinematic avatar. He met mentor von Trier over a game of Ping-Pong at the Danish Film School more than two decades ago, and is now a seasoned, internationally recognized commercial director with one previous feature film under his belt (*A Shot From the Heart* [1986]). Regarding the stringent Dogme strictures, he acknowledges the apparent irony of launching a cinematic manifesto at the end of the 20th Century. "The four of us [Vinterberg, Kragh-Jacobsen, von Trier and Levring] have very different points of view on that, but we aren't forcing anyone to work this way."

Levring laughs and notes, "Lars did ask Bertolucci to do one, but he said, 'I am too old to give my vow of chastity.' The reasoning behind this is quite strong though. These days there are no Bergmans, no Fassbinders; there are none of those people to lead the way. Films are being created by rote, and I think the actors especially suffer for this. Too

> "Lars did ask *Bertolucci* to do one, but he said, 'I am too old to give my VOW of CHASTITY.'"

often people talk about film in terms of, 'What's the target group?' This is appalling! It is terrible how few moving, original films are being made. I think Dogme is trying to counter that kind of think-

*Kristian Levring.*
photo by Eric Johnson

ing. I'm not saying that film shouldn't be a commercial venue, or that it's not a mass media. I'm okay with that. If you disagree, you should make books, or paintings.

"What matters," Levring adds, surveying the crowded city street, "is that you do your best to tell the story. For yourself, and for the people."

### Why has Dogme arisen in Denmark of all places?

I believe something quite special is happening in Denmark. Lars is one of the pioneers, but there is a lot going on there. I don't live there, I live in London now, so I'm not talking about myself. I think the Danish Film School is really good. People who go to film school always complain, but I think a lot of talent has been very well educated in that school. It has raised the country's pro-file…. Everywhere I go, film people are talking about Dogme. I think that the reason Americans are so interested is because they are so concerned with rules.

### It does sound puritanical and religious.

It is Dogme, after all.

### How did you become involved with Dogme 95?

I went to film school with Lars, and I also knew Søren from working in the film business. When he was doing his first film, I was like an assistant. Then when the whole thing started, they asked me to join it.

### The "Dogme brotherhood"—it makes you guys sound like the Masons or the Shriners—

We are not those kind of people. We are all after the '68 gener-ation, so we are just the opposite. It is very ironic that all of a sudden I have to sit and watch other people's movies and ask, "Does this follow the rules?" It is Dogme, it is not Dogme. What does that mean? Sometimes it is not possible to look at some-thing all together, specifically Jean-Marc Barr's film. There were some things that he did that we didn't agree with. We talked about it and he made changes. With Harmony, I think his film is very interesting. He's an interesting guy. But the whole idea of Dogme is that it's unfair to criticize or to tell you what I think the whole thing is about. At the end of the day, it is to be taken seri-ously, and I don't think it has been taken seriously enough.

### Do you view the Dogme rules as serious or playful?

There was an idea behind it—you can make films in different ways than one has been doing. Dogme proved that. And that is not irony. That is very important. The actual rules aren't ironic, although I think that the four of us are quite ironic in different ways. The sense of irony isn't in the rules. Like any rules—even the Ten Commandments—you can always interpret them. I made other rules for myself, such as, "I will shoot my film in continuity," which is a wonderful thing. I wouldn't do a shot in this film where the actors were not able to see each other, where the camera was covering up the other actors. That's not in the rules either, but I did these things because I felt it would make the film better. For instance, when they show it on German television and they dub a Dogme film, it's not a Dogme film and so forth. Every rule is open to interpretation. It says in the rules that the director must not be credited on the film. But what if he's credited on the poster...?

### That's pretty tricky.

The third commandment is you must not kill, but that doesn't mean you are not allowed to kill a moth. I know that's not very funny, but I think there are many ways to get around the rules, but not really. At the end of the day you can see if it's a Dogme film or not.

### There was some talk about changing the rules...

You can't change the rules. There was a thing in *Variety*. You cannot change the Ten Commandments. We can't; nobody can. It's not even within our power. If we changed them, it would be called something else.

### You can see how people might think the Dogme rules are a funny construct.

I can turn it around. When I talk to people they seem to get very mad about it. The other day, somebody came up and talked about a shot in Thomas' *Celebration*, which was not handheld. I said, "That shot is actually in Thomas' confession, but first of all, we like the film...." That's the most important thing—so I said, "Let's talk about that. Let's talk about whether that film would be different or better if it had not been shot as a Dogme film." I personally don't think it would've been as good a film as it is. If you want to do a Dogme film, go ahead. I don't think that any of us will ever do a Dogme film again. I think what Lars says is true. It's a cure. Do one and learn something from it, and bring some part of it to the next film. Personally, I think too many Dogme films are being made.

**Søren says he feels all the Dogme brothers have broken the rules by not shooting in 35mm, as the post-production transfer breaks one of the Dogme rules.**

In some way that's true. If you look at the rules, strictly shooting on video and transferring is not in the rules, but the film has to be 35mm as per the rules. We had a meeting about it, at Lars' house. We had ten or twelve of these dinners, and we decided to go for video because it would be easier. For me, video was fantastic. You can shoot so much—I shot 150 hours that was extra. Theoretically, you can talk about it not being Dogme—Søren is right—but we all agreed and accepted it.

**Isn't it ironic to launch a cinematic manifesto at the end of the 20th century?**

The four of us have very different points of view on that. I do agree that it is very ironic. For most of our generation, among those of us who like film, the golden age was the '70s, when there were a lot of things going on in the film business. In America, every year, there were two or three masterpieces—Altman, Scorsese, Coppola—all very original. But then I think it became much more of an industry, which means that there became a specific way of lighting or camera movement—and I know this because I have shot a lot of commercials and whenever you are in Beijing, Moscow, Los Angeles or Paris, you always end up shooting the same way. The reason it has become like that is because it's a way that producers can control a film.

"It is terrible how FEW moving, original films are being made. I think Dogme is trying to COUNTER that kind of thinking."

With Dogme, we are being serious about not shooting a film this way. I can say from shooting my film—because I shot it with English and American actors—that a lot of actors understand that Dogme is very important, because they are used to shooting films in a more traditional way. For them it was a big thing and they really liked it.

**Would you ever make another Dogme film?**

We talked about doing another one in fifteen years. I don't know if that's serious. I think that anyone who has made a Dogme film would use some parts of it again, but I think to do a second one becomes boring.

**Why did you go to Africa to shoot?**

You can do Dogme anywhere and I wrote the film for this specific location in Namibia, which is North of South Africa, and a big country. I had been there before and liked it. My reasons were purely practical. It is a country where you can get lost. There is also so much mystery to Africa.

**Far away from that "storm of technology" that
Lars von Trier speaks of in the manifesto?**

Actually, one of my fears, and I think for all four of us, is that Dogme will become some kind of producer's trick. And I think that's why when you talk to Lars he is so concerned about the irony. We worry that it will become just a new way to make cheap films.

**Did making a Dogme film transform you in the
way you expected?**

In a way. I am at the other end of the circle from Thomas. It had become more and more obvious to me that it was important to do things in a different way. I've been through all that. Søren said he was beginning to hate film, that he was losing his joy. And I think that is one of the most amazing things about Dogme. Thomas and Lars and then Søren talked about it, and I realize this is true, and I think all the actors in my film would say the same thing: Dogme is about joy. It's about enjoying what you are doing. I don't think we've had a more joyful shoot than our Dogme movies and I don't think the actors had a more joyful shoot. My film is very heavy— it's about dying, it's

<<<
*Henry (David Bradley) and Gina
(Jennifer Jason Leigh) in* The King
Is Alive.
courtesy of IFC Films.

about people going though big emotions—but it was still joyful. It's because when you shoot in that way, you don't spend ten hours on technology and two hours on content. When I did my film, I never thought of the Dogme rules as restrictions. Certainly there are restrictions, there always are when you do a film, but on the other hand there was so much liberty. Let's say you start nine in the morning. You're doing Scene 16, and you start rehearsing the scene and you tell you cameramen you're ready and you shoot for six hours and then go on the to the next scene. What does that mean? In a normal film, you would go in and light and do all these things and the actor has to go in and out of concentration. When we spend hours shooting something, the actors are in it from the start to finish, which allows them great concentration. It's a completely different way of working, without limitations or restrictions. It gives them bigger margins. In a "traditional" feature, I could never do more than one scene with an actor during the day, because they would be completely exhausted.

**You did a lot of improvisational work with the actors for *King*...**

But not during the film. We did a lot in rehearsal, two months before the shooting. Because Dogme is so much about character, it pushes you. You can't cheat when you get there.

**Filmmaking can be very isolating for a director. The Dogme community seems to have altered that.**

It's a big thing for me, and a big thing for all of us. Directing is a very lonely job. You very seldom meet other directors. Actors meet other actors, but there is usually only one director on a shoot. Meeting other directors, talking about how you work, how you arrive at things—this has been a big thing. Also, sometimes you meet other directors and you're not sure whether their intentions are good. Because we all wanted this Dogme thing to happen, there was never any kind of competition among the four of us.

**To make something so rarefied for the masses is very provocative.**

We talk about that all the time. There are so many people making Dogme rules that don't exist, but from the very beginning we talked about it being for audiences and not just an elite group of two people. It was not our intention to make it uncommercial. I was in Cannes, watching the first film, *The Celebration.* It was shown in the Palais [the festival's largest screening venue] to 6,000 people. All these respectable film people watching a film that was shot for about 500,000 pounds, on video, with no lights! And they were laughing! It was obvious they were really in this film. When it was important to be silent, they were silent, and at the end there was a standing ovation for at least fifteen minutes. I think Thomas merited that.

Secondly—this is a great lesson in film history—here you have a raw film, filmed in a very unconventional way, which goes against many, many industry precepts but it's still able to move a big crowd. For me Thomas' was the most important moment of Dogme. Not that there were all these famous people, but that there were human beings connecting. Film is *mass* media.

**What was the budget for this film?**

Mine was almost $3 million, which was a bit more than the others because it was shot in Africa, has twelve actors, and was financed with 70 percent American money through Good Machine in New York. Thomas' was $700,000; Lars' was $1 million and Søren's was $500,000.

**Those are very low figures. What has changed in regard to the commercial attention that has been given to your films?**

At the end of the day, a film is a product. When Søren, Lars and Thomas made their films, there was no interference by any producers in the story or in the way it was told. There were big concerns about those films—all the producers were talking about how they weren't going to make any money because they (the films) were too small. If you make a story about incest or about idiots, it's considered too narrow. The big difference is that they weren't thinking about a target group; they just made a film. And what they made was good and interesting and funny. Then of course, it becomes a product. But I'm okay with that.

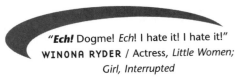

*"**Ech!** Dogme! Ech! I hate it! I hate it!"*
**WINONA RYDER** / Actress, *Little Women;*
*Girl, Interrupted*

## THOMAS VINTERBERG

"I am told that two people who saw the film fainted," Thomas Vinterberg, writer/director of *The Celebration*, fondly recalls. Winner of the 1998 Cannes Jury *The Celebration* is an unflinching portrait of a dysfunctional family reunion. "After they recovered, they went back and saw the rest of the film," he adds, smiling.

"I know it might sound a bit sadistic, but to me, it was a huge compliment." Incest, infidelity and suicide figure heavily in Vintenberg's tale of an affluent family gathered together to celebrate their patriarch's sixtieth birthday, and the director relates, "A lot of people asked if the story was based on my own experience. Most of it came from my imagination, I swear! My own family, I promise you, is very lovable. Though, I don't know what they would've done if I'd suddenly wept and confessed, 'Yes, yes! That is me.'"

To the outside eye, to so conspicuously return to the basics of filmmaking for *The Celebration*, especially in this tech-heavy age, appears unnecessarily rigorous and even a bit crazy. For Vinterberg, who previously made several award-winning shorts and the 1996 feature, *The Greatest Heroes,* the reason was completely pragmatic. "What is strange to me," says the director, "is that people don't see the obvious opportunities in it. The limitations of Dogme make it a very rich framework to work within."

Vinterberg's next ideological challenge arrived in the seductive envelope of Hollywood, and indeed, he was able to secure Claire Danes and Joaquin Phoenix to star in *It's All About Love*, an English-language drama. But the young director says he's wise to the game. "Greater possibilities are always tempting, but I don't think that will corrupt the way I make films. You can't create a good story simply because you have a lot of money. In my work, it is important to be committed to some sort of risk." He adds, "Not every film I make will be a Dogme film, but I found approaching a project in this way to be great fun, and very liberating." There is one problem, Vinterberg laughs, "It seems the idea scares people more than seduces them. At Cannes, Scorsese was very intrigued by the concept. I said, 'Join up! Jump over the barricades!' He laughed. Then he was drawn away by his bodyguards."

**The Dogme rules stipulate that a director is not
to be credited, yet you certainly relished coming
onstage to accept the prize at Cannes.**

That was my way of teasing my own monastery. I didn't understand anything, because I don't understand French at that speed,
especially coming from a model. I just heard my name, and the
rest was like an acid trip. The festivals are good and bad. It takes
me a long time to come back to earth after experiencing all these
things. I wasn't able to write for a long time.

**Did Lars send out invitations to other directors
to join Dogme?**

Yes, and he's not humble; he sent them to Kurosawa and
Bergman. What is very strange to me is that people don't see the
obvious opportunity in Dogme. Every painter has a frame to
work within. This is a very different frame, but the limitations,
the frame of Dogme, make it very creative to work within.

**The Dogme 95 Vow of Chastity—how did you
want people to view it?**

It is very funny and very serious at the same time. That was the
whole idea of it.

**You said you came up with it in an hour?**

The Vow of Chastity, yes, but the complete concept took a bit
longer. It was great fun, and really it was quite easy, taking the
conventions of filmmaking, and then forbidding them, one by
one. It was very liberating.

**What did it liberate you from?**

I felt stuck with a lot of ways of doing things. If you have to show
the emotional level of characters, you always you use the strings
to tell the stories of their lives, if you know what I mean, through
music and other means. So immediately when Lars told me his
idea I felt inspired by it. When I began, I didn't have any idea
about what film to make. The idea came very much out of The
Vow of Chastity. If you look at the Vow of Chastity before looking at the film, it looks quite difficult to make a film within those
circumstances, but it felt very good. It always takes around two
hours to make one shot, and so forth and so on. If you do film
or art that it is committed to some sort of risk, you must start on
a new level each time as much as you can. That way you challenge
yourself. I felt that the Dogme was a very precise, definite, and of

course, very funny way of doing it. It does ask a lot from the actors...we have this Dogme rule that says we're not allowed to move sound from one picture to another. So in all the cutaways under the speeches you would have to make the speech about forty-five times...that's a lot for an actor.

**What about the handheld camera rule—did you hold the camera much yourself?**

Not much. I didn't feel the need to. I had Anthony Dod Mantle [who shot on a Sony PC7 E], and he had assistants sometimes to hold other cameras; we sometimes had three. I felt that I was there to watch what was going on and I felt that what Anthony was doing was being one of the actors in a way, that his personality was a part of the film. I was there to regard what was going on.

**You use a lot of water imagery in the film.**

The title, the closing credit, the submerging in the bath...it's because in this film the sister drowns in a bathtub, so the sight of water is the thing that reminds us of her. Within the Dogme context it was quite difficult to make. We had to go to my house and use my kid's bathtub, and we had to make the title sequence a whole tune every time we did one title so we could cut into it. By that time we knew the film was going to Cannes. We stood there with our amateurish instruments and knew that this was going to be seen by Scorsese, and that was honestly quite scary.

**Why do you think *Celebration* moved people so much?**

It's difficult for me to understand...it's kind of unreal. To analyze why—it's very difficult. First of all, it's because I'm a genius! No, I'm kidding. The thing somehow clicks for people in Europe as well, and I experienced it in Denmark and travelling with the film. I think it's the clear cut impression of truth within the family—it's something that provokes people a lot; it's a part of everyone's life. The family as an institution is still very claustrophobic, but you can't avoid it, so it is a very vulnerable issue, so to speak, because it is unsolvable in some ways.

There is also a huge aggression in the film that somehow really appeals to other people's aggression, which worries me sometimes, but somehow the film also manages to deal with people loving each other. I don't have an answer. Do you?

**Perhaps because there is a human, unsolved
quality to the story, as well as in the shots...
many of which link up on a subliminal level.**

There is some truth to that. The film is about hiding more than
showing. This whole family is hiding away the truth and there is
only one person who is trying to view it. In a way, it's mechani-
cally what I did throughout the whole process of this film. There
are a lot of things that are difficult to see because it's hidden
behind the grain, or behind furniture, or other people. For
instance, if you have to communicate to an actor that he is supposed to be angry, the first thing you would ask him to do is hide
it. Pretend—come through the door and pretend that you are in
a smiley mood and just slam the door too hard. In hiding his
aggression, you get a feeling that there's something behind the
smile and that's the secret to every film, every film that works. If
you have two people making love on the stairs in the house, if you
see the whole scene, it's not in any way erotic, but if you walk a
little bit backwards and shoot through the banister, so you only
see a bit of the leg and the foot, you're hiding it. You start imagining what's happening behind that railing.... It's as simple as
that—it's constantly about hiding.

**Why isn't your next project a Dogme film?**

The whole idea was to make some kind of renewal. A repetition
of that would be very strange. That would be making a kind of
engine rather than creating something new.

**After *Celebration*, there has been a run of estab-
lished filmmaking rushing toward digital cinema.
How do you feel about that?**

It is a liberating thing. You have this weightless little camera that
captures everything you want and you can dispense with the huge
crews, the dollies and all the machinery. Suddenly, there is an
element of purity. I really enjoy the fact that it complements
filmmaking, that there is an alternative to this heavy machinery
which is the complete opposite. On *It's All About Love*, I am using
everything that is huge and heavy, the biggest cameras I can find.

**What filmmakers have inspired you?**

Coppola. It's not very original, but *The Godfather* is one of my
favorite films. I had that family structure in mind, as well as
Bergman's *Fanny and Alexander* for *Celebration*. I also adore Scorsese
and Truffaut.

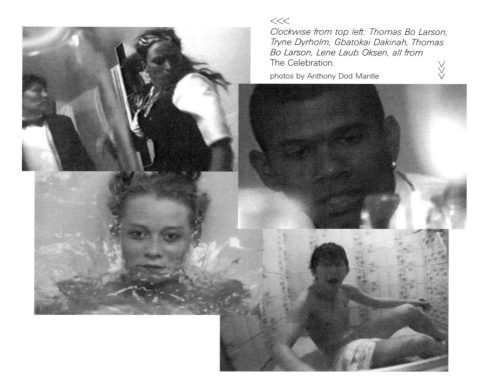

<<<
*Clockwise from top left: Thomas Bo Larson, Tryne Dyrholm, Gbatokai Dakinah, Thomas Bo Larson, Lene Laub Oksen, all from* The Celebration.

photos by Anthony Dod Mantle

### What did you want to be before you became a director?

I come from a pretty academic family. My father is a journalist and editor at a newspaper in Denmark and my older sister is an architect—but I wanted to be a rock star. I wanted to do something with a lot of glitter. It wasn't about being great, it was about being fast. I didn't have the guts to quit high school for music, so, frustrated that I couldn't compete with my friends, I started this filmmaking thing. I did this big project, which I started when I was sixteen, and that got me into the National Film School. In the end, the film turned out to be very bad, but at least it got me into film school.

### You have said doing a Dogme film is like going back to film school.

Yes, which was also what I needed. It was a fantastic experience. I felt very good making this film. It felt good being in the middle of that kind of community style of filmmaking. When I go back into things like lighting and continuity on this new film, I look forward to that because if I put up a lamp in the frame, there is a reason for it.

**What is your style of directing? Do you work with the actors emotionally like Lars?**

Normally, I would be more democratic and listen a lot, but sometimes I pretended it was a dialogue and at the end of the day I got what I wanted—that's the game it is. In this particular process, my method was to follow the method of the actor. For instance, the violent character, he's played by a fantastic improv actor, so I let him improvise; the person acting the father was very good at written dialogue and respects the written word, so he did the lines I gave him. There wasn't any specific, overall way.

**You went with the actors' overall bent then?**

It takes only five minutes to find out, and I consider them friends. It's nearly the same cast as *Greatest Heroes.*

**Why did you choose to do your new film, *It's All About Love*, as an English language film?**

The main reason is that I needed a change of scene. Getting out and exploring new territory is exciting. It also presents the possibility of creating on a larger scale. I am going to shoot on film. I never actually liked shooting on video, yet somehow I've become the president of this medium—though I consider myself merely its humble ambassador—and everywhere I'm presented as the "digital video camera guy." I've told everyone the reason we shot video was due to lack of money. When you have that kind of obstacle you have to use it, but I'm not that fond of it. On *Celebration* we used it because it fit with the aesthetic of that film. We used a one chip camera, where the image becomes very grainy and feels very organic, which is why I like it. Otherwise I find it a very difficult, very cold medium. Sure, you can do a lot with video afterwards, but if I make an image on film, and some technician says, "You could make the exact same image on a video camera," you'd have to work awfully hard to convince me.

"**I do think** film is an art form. All those tough-as-nails directors from the '30s and '40s who said they weren't making art were just being macho and pretentious. Of course, I understand the impulse to play it down and not get all artsy craftsy about it, but it's just as silly to say it's not an art. It's acting, writing, directing, lights and making all sorts of aesthetic decisions the whole time. What else would you call it? ❖ I don't think I'd shoot in DV until they make it look a little better. And when it comes to something like Dogme 95, *The Celebration* was great, but I wouldn't be restricted like that. Sometimes an overall idea of an aesthetic can be very helpful in guiding you creatively; if it's not, it's not worth anything. I guess sometimes when you espouse an artistic credo it can be very inspiring to people and I think it can also be intensely annoying."

**KENNETH LONERGAN** / Writer, *Gangs of New York,* writer/director *You Can Count on Me*

## What do you think about the "celluloid is dead" hue and cry?

I am curious to see if George Lucas can rekindle that sense of something organic from celluloid with these 24P HD cameras. I won't stop shooting on film until there is a very good reason to. It is still a very conservative art form and I think people will stick to the celluloid as long as they possibly can. In the meantime, the electronic medium has to compete and become very good. Digital filmmakers can show no sign of arrogance or people will jump back to celluloid.

## Do you think the Internet will become a useful tool for filmmakers?

To be honest, I use it is as a tool. I'm very practical. I do shopping, but I don't find the 'net very attractive or amazing. I'm just not too fascinated by it right now—it's too slow, and sitting down for hours and hours actually bores me a little bit.

## What's your new film about?

It's my own script with Morgens Rugov (co-writer of *The Celebration*) and it's a huge love story set in the future, but it's not sci fi.

## Does it have anything in common with the Godard film *Alphaville*?

We have almost the same point. It's a kind of portrait, or a warning about human life and society. For me, it's an effort beginning this project. My first rule was to avoid being repetitive, to avoid making another Dogme film so I said, "Okay! It has to be big! It has to be spectacular, and it has to be on film. This one I will over-storyboard, and my actors will not be allowed to improv! They will be like furniture!" Of course there will be improvisation. If the actor is not allowed to create life on screen, then there is no reason to make the film. I want to be consequential. I don't want to do anything that is mediocre illusion.

## Your actors are from the Hollywood pool. Have you been seduced by America?

To suddenly have access to bigger budgets and bigger possibilities is very tempting, but creating good stories is something you can't buy with money. I've been reading the scripts coming from the United States with great curiosity. Of course it is an important film center of the world, but sometimes with so much money, the stupidity of a project is completely ignored. That's very difficult to understand as a European. Here, in Europe, it's not an industry, it's not this mass product, and so very good things have come out of it. I came over to America once before, for a meeting after *Greatest Heroes*. I started talking about structure and plot points, but they wanted lyrical, European fancy stuff, no forward movement plot-wise, with lots of voiceover, and maybe in black and white. I felt very bored by that. I wanted to do something more American than the Americans wanted, which was very funny.

**How do you keep from compromising?**

There is always compromise whenever money and people are involved. I want to pick the reasonable compromise. I hate it though. It is such a big business and people are so responsible and so mature about what they are doing, which creates a lack of anarchy and courage. Without anarchy, there is no personality. You get a bunch of very reasonable, serious people walking around each other and never getting too drunk. It's boring to never make an idiot of yourself. We made idiots of ourselves with Dogme, which was completely ridiculous in its way, but it worked.

**What has if felt like being the poster boy for Dogme?**

Every time I talk to a person, outside my own small country, I get the feeling for what you are saying, and it's fantastic for me. My ego is big enough to begin with, but it kind of works for me because it creates a little bit of panic. What to do next? How to do it? I am not afraid of other people's judgement. It's an adventure to communicate so intimately with so many people.

**You must be really tired of talking about it.**

At some point a year ago, I just stopped talking about it and rejected any kind of interviews, closing the issue of Dogme. But on the other hand, to be honest, it's one of the things I'm most proud of. It has certainly changed me and the way I approach filmmaking.

Without Anarchy, there is no, personality.... It's boring to never make an idiot of yourself. We made IDIOTS of ourselves with Dogme, which was completely RIDICULOUS in its way, but it worked.

**When you are making a film, does it still feel like the beginning of an affair, an intangible excitement where anything can happen?**

> There's the belief that you must do what the audience wants, but there are feelings you must pursue as a filmmaker. It has to do with your purity towards the medium, because you lose that on your way. I try to not be repetitive with my work in order to be completely lost every time I start, so you get that feeling of being adventurous, almost suicidal, searching for something impossible, something unexplored. You can get that feeling of romance with the work or whatever you call it. It's a balance between using what you are good at while exploring something new. When you are repeating too many things in your work when it becomes claustrophobic and pathetic. It becomes a product. You know all the tricks to get where you need to, so it becomes a job. Success has nothing to do with what the audience wants, because we don't know what the audience wants.

**Has the way we view movies changed over the years?**

> The whole language changes every year, and film language is still the same but stylistically it changes, and within that the understanding of what happens on screen changes. I think the most revolutionary thing that has happened lately, in storytelling, is the beginning of the ironic film, the Tarantino wave. It's a kind of cynical filmmaking where things are not seriously meant. Everything is for fun and taking place in front of you. I saw this lecture with Paul Schrader and he talked about the idea of the antichrist film—that the moral of filmmaking, in modern film-making after Tarantino, instead of saving a child from being run over by a bus, you have the option to throw the child in front of the bus and people will still laugh and still love the character who does it because it's not meant seriously. It scares me a bit. To me, it's film losing power. People don't take it seriously anymore, which means nothing really matters. I think people will miss the meaningful, valid film, the film containing human life.
>
> If that is a genre, that is the kind of genre film I want to make.

# THE CONFESSION OF THOMAS VINTERBERG

As one of the DOGME 95 brethren and co-signatory of the Vow of Chastity I feel moved to confess to the following transgressions of the aforesaid Vow during the production of Dogme #1, *The Celebration*. Please note that the film has been approved as a Dogme work, as only one genuine breach of the rules has actually taken place. The rest may be regarded as moral breaches.

I confess to having made one take with a black drape covering a window. This is not only the addition of a property, but must also be regarded as a kind of lighting arrangement.

I confess to having knowledge of a pay raise that served as cover for the purchase of Thomas Bo Larsen's suit for use in the film.

Similarly I confess to having knowledge of purchases by Tryne Dyrholm and Therese Glahn of the same nature.

I confess to having set in train the construction of a non-existent hotel reception desk for use in *The Celebration*. It should be noted that the structure consisted solely of components already present at the location.

I confess that Christian's mobile or cellular telephone was not his own. But it was present at the location.

I confess that in one take, the camera was attached to a microphone boom, and thus only partially handheld.

I hereby declare that the rest of Dogme #1, *The Celebration* was produced in accordance with the Vow of Chastity.

Pleading for absolution, I remain
Thomas Vinterberg

# LARS VON TRIER

The spectacle of a forthright, unleashed human being following his or her creative hubris has always annoyed as many people as it's exhilarated. And now, standing under Cannes' blazing sun, Danish filmmaker Lars von Trier is uncomfortably, publicly, chawing on the blunt end of that conflicted excitement. Confronting his paralyzing fear of crowds for the sake of his new DV film, *Dancer in the Dark,* he warily leans against a balcony overlooking the Palais des Festival beach, facing the shouts and flashing cameras of a frenzied squadron of news crews hailing from three different continents. They all most definitely want to know how and why he crossed-wired the excesses of a farfetched D.W. Griffith melodrama with the 1950s Cinemascopic *joie de vivre* of a Gene Kelly musical. And from there, how he genomed his creation into an emotionally resonant morality fable set in 1960s rural America (a place he's never been and will never go to), scored by and starring Iceland's naïf pop-diva Björk (as Selma, a Czech factory worker slowly going blind), who twirls and warbles alongside the elegant French icon Catherine Deneuve

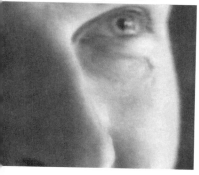

*Lars von Trier from* Lars *from 1-10.*
Courtesy of Shari Roman and Sophie Fiennes

(as Selma's best friend Cathy, a punch press operator), all of it unfolding spectacularly in front of 100 DV cameras. But the P.T. Barnum-like exuberance of von Trier's work is merely one small factor in the cineaste's larger filmmaking equation.

Regarded as one of Europe's most principled and iconoclastic auteurs, von Trier has had every one of his six feature films appear in the official program at Cannes. As fascinated as he is by culture (and others), however, he will not board an airplane. Not ever. He only recently moved from the three-story house he grew up in, to a new home not very far away. His childhood home; a comfortably bourgeoise domain replete with a large grassy backyard, a separate cottage that served as his home office, a carefully cultivated organic vegetable garden and a large playhouse, the province of his elder daughter from his first marriage. Hanging inside was a genial photo of another Danish icon, Hans Christian Anderson, who von Trier detests, calling him a celibate wanker. There are also trees on the property, which (it has been rumored) he used to practice "fire escapes," using a long rope that he invariably takes with him on his rare excursions.

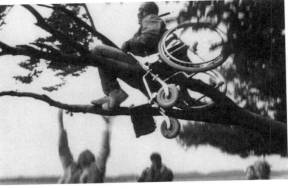

>>>
One of the idiots in a tree in The Idiots.
courtesy of Zentropa Productions

Having control, or being controlled, percolates through-out his work. "You can find all my anxieties in my films," von Trier says candidly. Rife with black humor and populated with characters who find themselves mentally, emotionally or physically impaired, his films show us characters whose inner natures are trapped as a battle rages among their intellect, spirituality and sexuality. In *Europa*, the lead character literally drowns in his own emotions. And Bess (played by Emily Watson) in *Breaking the Waves*, "the 'simple' girl in love who is dragged through heaven and hell by a wrathful God," as von Trier says, is another a case in point. And although his Bess howls at the sea, he himself is not adamantly against water, per se (as he loves kayaking). But when it came to moving locations for *Dancer in the Dark*, which was partially filmed in Sweden, across the Baltic Sea, near the Trollhattan forest, von Trier balked at the endless, churning vista and initially refused to board the boat. And when he went to Cannes for *Breaking the Waves*, he made half the journey, then turned around and went home. When traveling to Cannes for the premiere of *The Idiots*, he did so in an ancient camper that broke down on the way. Twice. But once there, he skewered his reputation as a dour perk-aesthete by lodging at the ultra-ritzy, cash-only Hôtel du Cap, showing he is capable of a cool irony, especially about himself, when stepping into the public eye. Even when speaking of his most commercially successful film to date, *Breaking the Waves*, he has opined, "For more intellectual audiences, the style will excuse the tears. The intellectuals will be able to permit themselves to cry because the story is so refined."

Notoriously moody, and wary of outsiders, von Trier likes to make an appearance on his own terms in his own good time. When we met for the Danish premiere of *The Idiots*, he arrived somewhat stiffly dressed in a tuxedo, always with one eye on an escape route. Back at his home base he was far more candid and relaxed—at least as much as he can be when confronted with a shopping list of intrusive, poking inquiry. "Contro is a key thing in my production and in my life, that's for sure," he says. The idea for the Dogme film aesthetic emerged from a desire to submit to the authority and rules he did not have as a child. Recalling his upbringing in a free-form, hippie-Marxist setting which he describes tartly as, "humanistic, cultural-leftist," von Trier consequently felt untethered, and deeply fearful. "Being too free is a lot of responsibility for a child. It gives you a lot of anxiety." He shrugs. "I don't think that there are a lot of people who don't have phobias to some degree, but to talk about it, especially to the degree I talk about it, I don't think is common." His fears increased a bit several years ago when his mother shocked him, on her death bed, by telling him that his father was not his father, "and that I was not really a Jew. She told me she had done this so that I could have more artistic genes…it was a very *Dallas* moment."

The mother who had given him his first Super 8 camera when he was ten years old, and the opportunity to pursue his passion, had lied to him. Von Trier shakes his head: "Not a Jew? Not to be part of the great 'victims' of the world? I was devastated." Von Trier wrote his visually stunning *Zentropa,* which unfolds like a night-

marish Shoah death dream, when he still believed he was Jewish. But he directed the film after the conversation with his mother. "I remember when I told this reporter from an Israeli paper, he cried, 'No! It's not true Lars. Say it's not true!' But, it was true. It was true."

After his mother's confession, von Trier decided to convert to Catholicism, and thereafter filmed

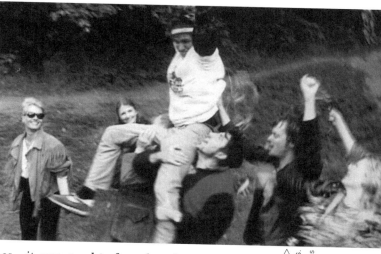

>> Triumphant idiots rejoice in The Idiots. courtesy of Zentropa Productions

his fiercely religious impassionata, *Breaking the Waves,* and created the canon for a religion he could use in his creative life, Dogme 95. A cleansing ritual. Asked if he would call Dogme a kind of cinematic high colonic, von Trier fixes me with a hateful look and barks, "Why do you ask these questions? These stupid questions. Why are you laughing? Is it the whiskey or are you nervous?" He straps his sandals back on and shakes his head. "These stupid questions you ask."

Before Dogme, von Trier was feeling strangled by options, by freedom. The color of a film always had to be just right. Scripts would take years to write. Actors were treated like props to be moved within a precise *mise en scene.*

But he longed for immediacy—the juicy, truthful moments that are born out of controlled chaos. But how could he give himself freedom without falling into the abyss? He would take on the role of both "higher power" and disciple, and construct a new universe.

With *The Idiots*, von Trier shot 80 percent of the film himself, using a miniDV camera, irrepressible enthusiasm and a raw emotional and visual aesthetic that many were unsettled by. The button-pushing storyline—young, smart, middle-class people pretending to be drooling simpletons into order to experience an alternate emotional truth—did nothing to soothe the mainstream.

If the *The Idiots* secured von Triers reputation as an iconoclast, his next film, *Dancer in the Dark,* confirmed his status as a world class digital provocateur. We meet again the day after the premiere of *Dancer* at a quiet table at the incredibly pricey, redolently peaceful Hôtel du Cap. Von Trier confesses in his softly accented English, continuing a conversation that began over a year ago, "I have this kind of perverse idea that I want to go into what was forbidden when I was child." He continues, "When I was growing up, my parents were not into films. I know they didn't like musicals. I do, especially the Gene Kelly ones. These images of America were really interesting to me. But they thought it was kind of superficial, and not true to what life was like. Melodrama, and religion too." He smiles enigmatically, perhaps musing over his own oeuvre. "They thought those were the worst."

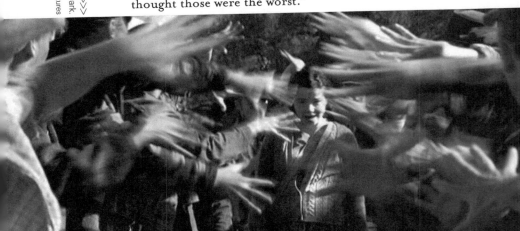

Up close, with his neatly shorn head, shapeless white T-shirt, pale trousers and passionately unrepentant stance, von Trier bears more than a fleeting resemblance to Joan of Arc, his favorite heroine/inspiration (at least as she's embodied in fellow countryman Carl Dreyer's masterpiece *The Passion of St. Joan*). And this is no mistake. Like von Trier, she's both a tempestuous visionary tormented for her beliefs, and a paradoxical concoction of cinematic invention, demanding egotism and wrenching emotional defenselessness. And like Dreyer, von Trier's cinematic dreams include staging a major trial by popular opinion.

But von Trier has other interests, too. "I was talking to a Danish writer, a good friend of mine," he continues, "who told me it was typical of my technique to split my personality into two or three of the female characters. That," he murmurs, "is an interesting idea." And characteristic of that underlying ethos, all of his films have captured the harsh irony inherent in redemption.

All have catapulted into the international mainstream of the Cannes Film Festival, too. Indeed, at the first screening of *Dancer*, the audience was decisively split; some were weeping uncontrollably, others were booing loudly. But von Trier—always rigorously, even perniciously honest about his conflicts and phobias—was not going to let a little personal divisiveness get in the way of his pleasure in the project, nor of the joy in seeing Björk named Best Actress, and especially, finally winning his long dreamt of prize, the Palme d'Or.

He asserts brazenly, "I hope there was booing. If everyone loved me and my film, I would feel I was at the end of my career. What is important for me," von Trier continues earnestly, "is to take a story like this, a story that if you hear it in words you would never accept it." He continues, noting that *Breaking the Waves* and *Dancer* tell essentially the same story, but in film, not in words. "If I can make you accept something in two hours and twenty minutes, then you have moved somehow, traveled someplace you thought you wouldn't go."

Von Trier has referred to *Dancer* as the finale to his trio [which includes Bess in *Breaking* and Karen in *The Idiots*] of sacrificial female films. "It is a trilogy in the sense that, more or less, I've made three films with the same female lead, a strong character, sacrificing herself," he says candidly. "But it's nothing I do on purpose. Part of the reason for this comes from my father. When he wanted to be really sarcastic, he would say something about a 'Golden Heart,' [the title of a series of children's books about a girl with a saintly heart]. But I also just found out today another reason why I do these women: When I was seven years old, I got a projector and I asked my uncle [who is a documentary film-maker] for something to show on this 16mm thing, and he gave me something that had been thrown out...and this was, by chance, the trial of Joan of Arc [Dreyer's *The Passion of St. Joan*], which I must have watched 1000 times. I've been brainwashed. What else could you expect?"

And what about the public *sturm und drang* between actor and director? (Björk, infuriated with the emotional manipulation von Trier often uses to help his performers move into their characters, reputedly stormed off the set several times, later returning to shred von Trier's T-shirt with her teeth on one occasion. Von Trier in turn, shortly before the festival, helpfully referred to his star as a "madwoman.") In response to the question, von Trier says enthusiastically, "We did have some crises, but we also have had a fantastic contact. I must say that this work with Björk has been very rewarding. I was shooting with this DV camera on my shoulder, and in this way I can get physically close to the actors. I do all kinds of cheap tricks, tell jokes and touch the actors and get really, really close. And Björk is so clever, I can get this close and she responds so quickly...which is all good, but also can be really evil. This scene where Björk is killing the man and she is in a terrible state and she obviously feels it. I remember saying to her, 'You have to kill him, he's suffering, he's suffering!' Then afterwards saying, 'Look at him! You've just killed your best friend!' You have to be extremely sadistic, but this is because it is part of the work." He pauses, "Yeah, well maybe then I'm not enough of a real sadist. It was not nice."

Although the relationship between star and director did seem on the mend when the pair arrived together at the ceremony and von Trier opined in his acceptance, "Though I know she doesn't believe me, if you meet her, tell her I love her very much," all is not yet forgiven. Von Trier offers ingenuously, "What can I say? She is not an actor, which is a surprise for me, because she seems so professional. But that is what is so good about the whole thing. She is not acting, she is feeling everything, which is also extremely hard on her. And extremely hard on everyone else. I worked like a hangman, in the sense that I was the one to put her [in that state] all the time, but maybe the biggest problem is, we understand each other so extremely well. It's almost like a sexual thing because we've been so close." He adds hastily, "We haven't had sex! But now it's kind of this divorce feeling. I'm sure at a certain point she will come out and say she is ready to talk about all this. In maybe ten, twenty years. But as I see it now, it is the only way it could be." Björk for her part has pronounced her permanent retirement from acting.

Deneuve, who knows her way around a pointed cue or two, says her excursion into von Trier's filmmaking world wasn't nearly as truculent. "But it is one of the most unusual experiences I have ever had," she says. "I never had a director so physically close, with no technicians around. And once we had read the scenes, he wanted us to break the lines and try to improvise," an exercise Deneuve had "never attempted, certainly not in a foreign language. It always gave more possibility...to everything," she says, "and I felt a great freedom this way. I was scared, yes, but he is someone, even though he is very shy, who is very good at making people at ease, because he feels so sure, so secure about what he is doing."

Good friend and *Breaking the Waves* lead Stellan Skarsgård (who played the tormenting husband to Emily Watson's saintly Bess), points out reasonably, "Lars is a very sweet man, but all directors are control freaks." He continues, "And technically, yes, he is one of the best filmmakers in the world. But if you look at his early films, they're like stainless steel. Perfect and ice cold. *Europa* was created at home at his desk, all him and no input, no irrationality, no idea that was not his. Things used to go from the storyboard directly to the camera, which was good to look at, but boring. And when he began shooting, he

**"Lars wanted** us to improvise within the [construct] of the scenes. Once we had done the scenes, he wanted us to break the lines and try to give more realistic and more natural behavior within the scene. I felt a great freedom...I've never worked that way before and I don't think many have. Lars is quite special. I have had very unusual experiences with directors, but I never had a director with no technicians around, speaking, being so close physically to the actors. With Lars, usually the camera is there, very intimate, with no lights. As for those 100 cameras that he used in the dance sequences, yes, that is a lot of work for them, for the technicians, but not for us. You never saw the technicians; it was very mysterious. We would rehearse and prepare and sometimes the cameras were behind the bench, behind a coat, on the floor, just behind a foot. It was incredible. With von Trier, we didn't rehearse; sometimes we just shot. He would have the camera on one shoulder. Even in those scenes with 100 cameras, he always had his camera on his shoulder. The thing is, sometimes you don't know what you've been doing, you don't know where the scene is going. You feel like you have no idea of the peak of the whole scene, but you have to accept that. You have to trust him. It's really all about trust."
**CATHERINE DENEUVE /**
Actress, *Dancer in the Dark*

said to the crew, 'If you find one image in that film that is not in my shooting script, I will give you a bottle of whisky.' It is very brave to have so much success, with so many perfect pieces and just let go of it. He had the courage to totally change his way of working so dramatically because he wants to get something more out of it. Now, he is letting chaos happen and still molding it into something." [No one was able to claim the whiskey.]

This new confluence of emotion and technology all agree, comes from the Dogme. One rule in particular—that the camera must be handheld—certainly helped von Trier to be more fluid on the non-Dogme *Dancer*. It also made it all the more possible for him to have more contact with the actors, instead of just looking at the monitor and shouting at them. With *Dancer*, there was nothing but the actors and their talent, the director, and the story. Nobody could hide behind anything, and there were no excuses. The process does make him more vulnerable, he knows, but it's also undeniably seductive, and it's given him a lot more freedom to create.

Von Trier proffers his own analysis: "I think it's because I'm getting older, and I am beginning to understand that there might be other people in the world who could contribute something. I'm not the only one who knows about everything. I don't know what I would've done with Björk in *Element of Crime*, for example. She could've been standing in a corner screaming," he drawls, "and then I would've panned away from her."

But despite all these artistic strides, von Trier hasn't completely released himself from all of the heavy stones that keep him earthbound. "For instance...flying," he says tugging unconsciously at the scarf knotted around his neck. "No, no, honestly, I think even if I could fly I would be too scared to go to the States. It's big and it seems very unsafe. Especially the cities. But I'm sure there are a lot of places I would love. There is a lot of beautiful nature and also nice people who don't have this big KKK hood on...." He laughs, and points out sweetly, "I've seen a lot of films about America...you shouldn't underestimate that, but even so, I prefer fiction. And I would also like to say, Kafka wasn't there either and he made a great book about it [*Amerika*], which is where, I am sure, I have gotten all my knowledge of your country. And, finally, I would also like to quote Ingrid Bergman on this: 'Of course we never went to Casablanca.' It's a film. That is what it is. It's fake. It's all fake."

# DOGME FILMS TO DATE

Dogme #1: *Festen* (Denmark)
Directed by Thomas Vinterberg
Produced by Nimbus Film Productions
Avedøre Tværvej 10
DK-2650 Hvidovre
Denmark
Phone: (+45) 36 34 09 10
Fax: (+45) 36 34 09 11
Link: www.dogme95.dk

Dogme #2: *Idioterne* (Denmark)
Directed by Lars von Trier
Produced by Zentropa Entertainments
Avedøre Tværvej 10
DK-2650 Hvidovre
Denmark
Phone: (+45) 36 78 00 55
Fax: (+45) 36 78 00 77
Link: www.dogme95.dk

Dogme #3: *Mifunes Sidste Sang*
(Denmark)
Directed by Søren Kragh-Jacobsen
Produced by Nimbus Film Productions
Avedøre Tværvej 10
DK-2650 Hvidovre
Denmark
Phone: (+45) 36 34 09 10
Fax: (+45) 36 34 09 11
Link: www.dogme95.dk

Dogme #4: *The King Is Alive* (Denmark)
Directed by Kristian Levring
Produced by Zentropa Entertainments
Avedøre Tværvej 10
DK-2650 Hvidovre
Denmark
Phone: (+45) 36 78 00 55
Fax: (+45) 36 78 00 77
Link: www.dogme95.dk

Dogme #5: *Lovers* (France)
Directed by Jean-Marc Barr
Produced by TF1 International
125 Rue Jean-Jacques Rousseau
92138 Issy-Les-Moulineaux
France
Phone: (+33-1) 41 41 15 04
Fax: (+33-1) 41 41 31 76

Dogme #6: *julien donkey-boy* (USA)
Directed by Harmony Korine
Produced by Independent Pictures
42 Bond Street
New York, NY 10012
USA
Phone: (+1) 212 933 1200
Fax: (+1) 212 993 1201

Dogme #7: *Interview* (Korea)
Directed by Daniel H. Byun
Produced by CINE 2000 Production
Foreign sales representative: MIROVI-SION Inc.
7F. Garden Yeshikjan B/D, 45-18
Youido-dong,
Yongdungpo-gu, Seoul 150-010
Korea
Phone: (+82) 2 375 2567/9
Fax: (+82) 2 737 1185

Dogme #8: *Fuckland* (Argentina)
Directed by Jose Luis Marques
Produced by ATOMIC FILMS S.A.
Castillo 1366 (1414) Buenos Aires
Argentina
Phone: (+54) 11 4771 0400
Fax: (+54) 11 4771 6003
Link: www.fuckland.com.ar

Dogme #9: *Babylon* (Sweden)
Directed by Vladan Zdravkovic
Produced by AF&P, MH Company
Sveavaegen 4
85239 Sundsvall
Sweden
Phone: (+46) 60 14 84 54
Mail: vladan@ite.mh.se

Dogme #10: *Chetzemoka's Curse*
(USA)
Directed by Rick Schmidt, Maya
Berthoud,
Morgan Schmidt-Feng, Dave Nold,
Lawrence E. Pado, Marlon Schmidt
and Chris Tow.
Produced by FW Productions
P.O. Box 1914
Port Townsend, WA 98368
USA
Mail: lightvideo@aol.com

Dogme #11: *Diapason* (Italy)
Directed by Antonio Domenici
Produced by FLYING MOVIES s.r.l.
Via del Governo Vecchio 73
00186 Roma
Italy
Phone: (+39) 06 6813 6673-4
Fax: (+39) 06 6813 6675
Co-producer: Minerva Pictures
Via Domenico Cimarosa 18
Roma
Italy
Phone: (+39) 06 85 43 841
Fax: (+39) 06 855 8105
Mail: minervai@tin.it
Link: www.minervapictures.com
Link: www.rarovideo.com

Dogme #12: *Italiensk For Begyndere*
(Denmark)
Directed by Lone Scherfig
Produced by Ib Tardini Zentropa
Entertainments
Avedoere Tvaervej 10
2650 Hvidovre
Denmark
Phone: (+45) 36 86 87 88
Fax: (+45) 36 86 87 89

Dogme #13: *Amerikana* (USA)
Directed by James Merendino
Produced by Gerhard Schmidt and Sisse
Graum Olsen
Cologne Gemini Filmproduktion and
Zentropa Productions 2
Avedoere Tvaervej 10
2650 Hvidovre
Denmark
Phone: (+45) 36 86 87 88
Fax: (+45) 36 86 87 89

Dogme #14: *Joy Ride* (Switzerland)
Directed by Martin Rengel
Produced by ABRAKADABRA FILMS AG
Theaterstrasse 10
CH-8001 Zürich
Swiss
Phone: (+41) 1 254 58 90
Fax: (+41) 1 262 45 14
Mail: abrakadabra@swissonline.ch

Dogme #15: *Camera* (USA)
Directed by Rich Martini
Produced by Rich Martini
P.O. Box 248
Santa Monica, CA 90406
USA
Mail: richmartini@yahoo.com

Dogme #16: *Bad Actors* (USA)
Directed by Shaun Monson
Produced by Nicole Visram
Immortal Pictures
4000-D West Magnolia Blvd.
Suite 260
Burbank, CA 91505
USA
Link: www.badactors.net

Dogme #17: *Reunion* (USA)
Directed by Leif Tilden
Produced by Kimberly Shane O'Hara
and Eric M. Klein
5460 White Oak Avenue E335
Encino, California 91316
USA
Phone: (+1) 818 461-8929
Fax: (+1) 818 416 8933
Mail: yelduck@aol.com
Link: www.reunion81.com

Dogme #18: *Et Rigtigt Menneske*
(Denmark)
Script and Director: Åke Sandgren
Produced by Ib Tardini
Zentropa Productions
Avedoere Tvaervej 10
2650 Hvidovre
Phone: (+45) 36 78 00 55
Fax: (+45) 36 78 00 77
Mail: Lizette.gram@filmbyen.com

Dogme #19: *Når Nettene Blir Lange*
(Norway)
Directed by Mona J. Hoel
Produced by Malte Forssell
Freedom From Fear A/S
Mail: maltefilm@euromail.se

Dogme #20: *Strass* (Belgium)
Directed by Vincent Lannoo
Produced by Dadowsky Film
Rue De Belgrade 13
1190 Forest (Brussels)
Belgium
Phone 0032 2 538 55 71
Mail: radowsky.films@online.be

Dogme #21: *En Kærlighedshistorie*
(Denmark)
Directed by Ole Christian Madsen
Produced by Bo Ehrhardt, Birgitte Hald
and Morten Kaufmann
Nimbus Film Produktion ApS
Avedøre Tværvej 10
DK-2650 Hvidovre
Denmark
Phone: (+45) 36 34 09 10
Fax: (+45) 36 34 09 11
Mail: dogme@nimbusfilm.dk

Dogme #22: *Era Outra Vez* (Spain)
Directed by Juan Pinzás
Produced by Pilar Sueiro
ATLÁNTICO FILMS, S.L.
Plaza Conde Valle Suchil, 15
28015 Madrid
Spain
Phone: (+34) 915 931 781
Fax: (+34) 915 931 780
Mail: atlanticofilms@wanadoo.es

Dogme #23: *Resin* (USA)
Directed by Steve Sobel
Produced by Steve Sobel
Organic Film
1966 North Beachwood Drive #12
Hollywood, CA 90068
USA
Phone: (+1) 323 464-1271
Mail: resin@anet.net
Link: www.resin-themovie.com

Dogme #24: *Security, Colorado* (USA)
Directed by Andrew Gillis
Produced by Andrew Gillis
Grammar Rodeo LTD
128 S. Churchill Dr.
Fayetteville, NC 28303
USA
Phone: (+1) 910 484-9828
Mail: grammarrodeo@hotmail.com,
andygillis@aol.com

# DOGME CERTIFICATE FORMULA

Original title: ...........................................................................................................

Title in English: ........................................................................................................

Nationality: ...............................................................................................................

### Sworn statement

In regard to my feature film " ............................................................ " I hereby solemnly swear that
I have adhered in full to the Dogme95 Manifesto and the Vow of Chastity. I thus request
that a dogme certificate be issued and forwarded.

.............................................            .......................            .............................
Director's signature                          Date:                      Place

Production Company:
(Name/address/phone/fax/E-mail)

Foreign sales representative:
(Name/address/phone/fax/E-mail)

Director:

Screenplay & Dialogue:

Director of Photography:

Producer:

Name of the Part:                                              Main Cast:

..................................................     =     ..................................................

..................................................     =     ..................................................

..................................................     =     ..................................................

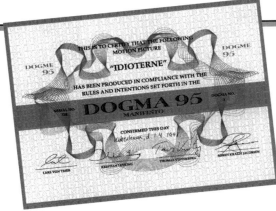

Budget in US dollars:

Length in minutes:

By this I confirm my willingness to pay Danish Kroner 10.000 for the Dogme 95 Certificate.

.............................................................................
(Director's signature)

Since this feature film has a fair- to high budget I volunteer to pay Danish Kroner 30.000 for the Dogme 95 Certificate.

.............................................................................
(Director's signature)

By this I ask for an annulment of the demand for a payment of Danish Kroner 10.000 for the Dogme 95 Certificate (Please state your reasons for an annulment):

.............................................................................................................................................................

.............................................................................................................................................................

.............................................................................................................................................................

.............................................................................................................................................................

.............................................................................................................................................................

.............................................................................................................
(Director's signature)

When I have finished the film and received the Dogme certificate I agree to send a VHS copy of the film (preferably with English subtitles) to the Dogme Secretariat to be filed in the Dogme archives.

.............................................................................
(Director's signature)

Send to: Nimbus Film, Dogme Secretariat, Avedoere Tvaervej 10, DK-2650 Hvidovre, Denmark

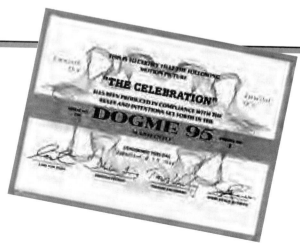

On *TimeCode:*

"When I did Mike Figgis' *TimeCode*, I didn't care whether it turned out to be good film or not, the process was going to be fun. You synch up your watches, you go and you have a take and no one can or is allowed to say, 'Cut!' That's total freedom. After a while you get the endorphin rush you get when you do live theater. You don't normally get that in movies because there's so much preparation. It was great fun. The biggest threat to what I am doing, or what most actors are doing, is fear, because it's absolutely natural to be frightened when you get in front of the camera. Yet fear blocks you and shrinks you. Abilities like professionalism, brilliance and skill...those things are very secondary, they can actually be a hindrance. To a certain degree skill and elegance are antithetical to life. When everything is polished and shiny like stainless steel, it can reflect life, but it is isn't life. I am, after forty-five plus films, very skilled technically. I can hit a mark blindfolded but I try not to. I try constantly to muck up my performance. I'm not good at improvisation, but doing something like the Figgis film messes up my performance in a nice way, and then the irrationalities that you carry around inside begin to pop out and suddenly everything you do becomes alive."

On Lars von Trier:

"I was supposed to have a much larger role in *Dancer in the Dark.* Lars called me when I was at my old summerhouse with a veranda, near the Baltic Sea. Actually, I was in the outhouse and I got a call from Lars, and he says, 'Can you sing, can you dance?' and I said, 'I can't sing, but you can fix that digitally, can't you? And I'm not really a dancer but I can move to music.' 'Okay,' he says, 'I'll write a singing and dancing role for you.' Then I had all these other conflicts, promises I had made to other films, and they were in conflict with *Dancer,* so Lars found another role for me, but I couldn't do that one either. So I ended up coming down to Copenhagen for two lines. Then he said, 'You weren't very good, I'll probably cut you out,' but as it stands, I'm still in the movie. ❖ I know how it sounds, but if you like people it can be quite entertaining to constantly insult each other. It's very European. When Lars is mad, he is not really mad; though sometimes he can be a hypersensitive, over-intelligent child. *The Idiots* is not a good or a bad film, but it's not entertainment, either. When I saw it at Cannes, I was very disturbed throughout the film. I didn't know whether I liked it or not. It was very brave and strange and brutal. Very upsetting, and very imperfect. Which is very interesting, as Lars, technically, is one of the best filmmakers in the world. ❖ When I first saw *Element of Crime* I said, 'Wow, I'd like to work with this director.' When he came to *Europa* (*Zentropa* in the States), it was like stainless steel to me, perfect and ice cold. And when he did that, he did all that at home at his desk, without any irrationality, no input, not one idea that was not his. ❖ All directors are control freaks, and Lars is as well. But he is talented enough to realize he can control chaos. He lets chaos happen and still molds it into something."

On Hollywood:

"The first time I was invited to a Hollywood party—well, I'm a Swede, we know how to party— and I rolled up my sleeves and prepared for a long night and I came to realize that we had been invited but we weren't really wanted. And before I finished my second drink, everyone was gone—the party lasted an hour. I rolled down my sleeves, went back to my hotel and got drunk in my room."

**STELLAN SKARSGÅRD** / Actor, *Breaking the Waves, TimeCode,*
*Signs & Wonders, Dancer in the Dark*

# LIGHTS CAMERA DIGITAL ACTION!

## DPs AT WORK

In counterpoint to the old school style of filmmaking where shaky camerawork is verboten, the handheld DV camera careens about within the frame, an intentionally technical technique of moving the camera to convey activity.

During the 1970s, *vérité* mannerisms became commonplace and were eventually superseded by the invention of the Steadicam, all but vanishing from the screen for a while. When used with prudence, they can affect an uncommonly brutal realism, as well as an emotional interplay in which the cinematographer becomes a performer in the action. DP-turned-director Haskell Wexler's 1969 *Medium Cool* is an early, prescient example of *vérité* politics, George Romero's pioneering horror flick *Night of the Living Dead* was made the same year, and 1970's *What Do You Say to a Naked Lady?* transferred Alan Funt's voyeuristic (but previously G-rated) "candid camera" to the big screen with X-rated results.

The hands-on approach, emerging from a desire to break with the heavyweight hardware of 35mm and achieve greater freedom of movement, enables cinematographers who take up DV to move in step with the action around them. In terms of craft, it provides a fluidity of movement and execution, with far less time required for set-ups during filming.

Aesthetically buoyant, even with the most stygian storyline, the speed of the image capture DV presents, plus the portability of the smaller cameras, offers new means of expression for DPs, allowing them to capture movements and angles that would be impossible under conventional means. With an instinct for the texture of light, color and image, they create their lighting from natural elements, or by using elegantly simple set ups to convey that naturalism, reinforcing the impression of real life. The one disadvantage in utilizing existing light, especially on Dogme films, is less definition and a lack of clarity which can make the video grain more visible. The stark homeliness of the DV aesthetic, though lacking the lush palette of 35mm, compensates for its shortcomings with a visceral dignity, an unsettling visual honesty and the gloriously dark beauty of reality.

## ( MARYSE ALBERTI )

"All my life, all I've wanted to do is travel, to have extraordinary experiences," says Maryse Alberti, who swears it was "sheer luck" that she fell into cinematography. "When I came to visit America at nineteen, the only intention I had was to have a good time, and to take photographs," she says. "I had no big life plan. I come from a village in the South of France where the best that is expected of you is to become a schoolteacher."

Education's loss is cinema's gain. The forty-seven-year-old cinematographer, who currently lives in New York's Tribeca with her husband and seven-year-old son, has come to be regarded as one of the most respected DPs working in independent film today. This is due in part to her unerring eye, a slate of stunning yet wildly divergent films, and an almost uncanny ability to bring a project's very essence to the screen.

This visualist's wild ride first began when Alberti, who was looking for a way to make some extra cash, took a job shooting stills on a porn movie for $25 dollars day. "Everybody seems to know this about me," she laughs unashamedly. Taking the assignment, Alberti got bit by the film bug, and it altered her life forever.

Alberti began her film career on low budget documentaries, with projects like *H-2 Worker* (1989) about Jamaican farm hands; *Crumb* (1994), which delves into the off-

kilter world of cartoonist R. Crumb (both films won awards at the Sundance Film Festival for best cinematography); and the stellar Oscar® winner *When We Were Kings* (1996), about the life and times of boxing legend Muhammad Ali. Alberti's initiation into the world of independent feature filmmaking came in the form of writer-director Todd Haynes (who Alberti dubs a "brilliant imagist") and producer Christine Vachon (Killer Films), who asked the budding lenser to take on Haynes' debut feature, *Poison* (1991). She followed that utterly original film with Anthony Drazan's *Zebrahead* (1992), a lyrically gritty look at urban racial tensions. And in the equivalent of a rousing cinematic double-header, Alberti went on to shoot two of 1998's most diametrically opposed and provocative features: Todd Solondz's *Happiness* (1998), a tightly crafted and hypnotically restrained story about pedophilia which nabbed the Critics' Prize at the Cannes Film Festival, and Haynes' *Velvet Goldmine* (1998), which dazzles with fantastical color washes in its stunning recreation of London's 1970s glam rock era, which earned a 1999 Independent Spirit Award for cinematography. All in all, this sensational filmography is not

"I look at Gordon Willis (*Manhattan*) a bad start for someone who never intended to go into filmmaking.

who is fantastic, or Bob Richardson (*Natural Born Killers, Casino*), whom I consider to be revolutionary—I am so inspired by them," says Alberti, who tends to find her ideas through visceral exploration and instinctive energy.

Alberti demurs gracefully when asked about her own style, claiming, "I am still not sure whether I have a style. I started so late, when I was around thirty, and I've only done seven dramatic features." She hesitates, and adds more strongly, "I actually don't think DPs should have a style, per se. I think they should have taste. And sure, I have things I like in the way of color and light. But I also think that style is a joint effort, involving the script and the director."

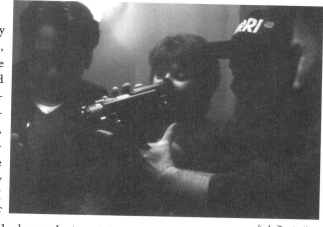

(l to r) Robert Sean Leonard, cinematographer Maryse Alberti, director Richard Linklater and Ethan Hawke prepare a shot for Tape.

courtesy of Lions Gate Films

Following this ethos, she worked closely with actor and director Stanley Tucci (*Big Night*) on *Joe Gould's Secret* (1999). Alberti used a monochromatic palette to provide the essential touch for this quintessential small film. The 1940s set piece tells the quirky, true-life tale of New Yorker magazine scribe Joe Mitchell (played by Tucci) and his unusual friendship with the flamboyant Joe Gould (Ian Holm), a bohemian writer who claimed to be penning the oral history of the world.

She also utilized those talents on Richard Linklater's DV feature, *Tape*, a tightly wound memory piece starring Ethan Hawke, Uma Thurman and Robert Sean Leonard, which bowed at Sundance 2001. Set completely within the confines of a seedy motel room, Alberti's style here is stripped down, tightly focused and fiercely electric. Her handheld camera emerging as the unseen fourth, equally powerful player in this modern-day masochism tango.

Despite her meteoric rise—or perhaps because of it—Alberti feels that the only way to keep developing as an artist is to stay open to other forms of creation. "Picasso said that it takes a lifetime to learn how to draw like a child," she notes. "I think as you grow in your craft, it becomes harder and harder to find that pure zone of creativity. You try to bring that to your work, but on a film set, it's quite impossible. They are ready and waiting for you, and you still have to go...even if you're not quite there. When it's an hour later, and you go, 'I know!' it's too late. That's when it's really tough."

**You started off as a still photographer, didn't you?**

I was thirty years old when it happened, and it just began to take off. I had no connections in the film world. But it makes a lot of sense...you are still working with film, light and frame. The only difference is that it's moving. You tell a story in two hours with pictures. For one photo, I make it alone in my studio while in a film I make it with 100 people in forty days. It's a whole different thing. But it's still a joy, absolutely. It's a great thing to work in the studio by yourself where it's all about the creative process. On a film set, the trick is to preserve a little bit of the creative process, amidst the concerns of money, time, personalities...that's the trick—to keep the vision.

**What is your still work like?**

I photograph people and places. I mix images. I use Plexiglas. A lot of my images are about colors and shapes. I do it for pleasure. But I've always done artwork. I've never made a lot of money doing it, though.

**How did you end up as a DP?**

I fell by accident into the film industry. I live in the East Village and my world is a world of artists. So I met the right people, and the woman who did *H-2 Worker*, Stephanie Black, we met and clicked and she didn't have a lot of money. We were young and crazy and took a lot of risks. Sleep on the ground, get arrested by the police every other day.... I don't think I could do that again.

**How did you end up shooting your first feature?**

I met Todd Haynes and Christine Vachon a long time ago at a company called Apparatus. It was a small company that produced short films. And someone I knew from the art scene was going to do a short film for them. And through this I met Todd and Christine. I shot a very short film for her. And Todd had this script called *Poison* and we liked each other a lot and he gave me a chance. It was a time when I was younger. You never know what you're getting into when you begin something.

## How do you approach your work?

I work a lot by instinct—I don't have a formula. As a cinematographer, I know a certain amount of technique. But sometimes you just follow your feelings. Once, I went to listen to a talk by Vittorio Storaro where people where asking about his methods, what gel he used, which filters, but instead he just started talking about the moon, and the sun, the conscious and the unconscious. What I learned from that is that you must learn your craft but don't let it be the element that rules you. Trust your intuition and instincts instead. In that way, *Velvet Goldmine* was an exercise in excess, while *Happiness* was an exercise in restraint. I tried to be very naturalistic, very bare. I tried to get rid of all the ornamentation the photographer sometimes uses in a film, when you have this tendency to make things look good, pretty. Especially after *Velvet Goldmine* I was ready to be very stark. The story was so strong so I felt the cinema should be very restrained.

## What do you think of working in DV?

I think it's very exciting to work in these new pictures, but it's all how you use it. Look at early video artists like Nam June Paik and Bill Viola. What I hope is that this new tool frees film from always having to tell the story so it can be used for more abstract images like painting. A painter can choose to work with acrylics, oils or pastels. It's getting so that filmmakers can use different films and textures. Things that have that forbidden element in our culture are very interesting to me. Working that way, one can be more voyeuristic, more than an exhibitionist. So the camera is perfect. Does the size of the camera foster more handheld images?

One can work handheld using one of the smaller 16mm cameras, which is great for documentaries. I really like an Aaton, which is very nice, very light. I did a lot of handheld work on *Crumb* and *H-2 Worker*. It's very small and people don't notice it after a while. When I work on a documentary, I find that I am more in charge, because you have to take in things as they happen. When I shoot in 35mm, I don't really feel as close to the camera. It's too big, too much of a separate thing.

## Do you think that working in DV gives you more of an intimacy with the actors?

Working with the actor is the job of the director. I try to make actors as comfortable and make them look good or bad as the script and the director call for.

## What inspires you?

I try to go look at many different art forms. For my own pleasure, I still take photographs. I go to look at dance, theater, music—all kinds of performances. When I work in documentaries, sometimes I find myself emotionally influenced by an image. I might go and see a piece by Laurie Anderson; I took my son to see a Nam June Paik show at the Guggenheim, which he loved. Jackson Pollack...it's all good. Good art is good for the soul. I might even go into a store in South America and see this grim fluorescent light in the back, with a yellow light on the side and think, "Hey, that looks great. That's a good idea." I think common, everyday occurrences, along with every art form, all have the potential to inspire you.

## Is your work the most important thing in your life?

If you had asked me that a few years ago I would've said yes. But now that I have a little boy, he is the main importance in my life. I had been asked to shoot *Boys Don't Cry* and *American Psycho* but I didn't want to leave him. I think in a way, that's really healthy. I think that it's good to think about what is essential in life and find that it is actually quite simple. I don't really need that many things. I have all the things that are essential to me. All the fame, glory and money are great. If you get it, great. If you don't, that's okay too. I love spending time with my son, and right now, he still wants to spend time with me. In this way, perhaps I have made choices that have been bad for my career, but good for my life.

## How did you end up shooting Rick Linklater's *Tape*?

I met Rick two years ago. We were on the dramatic jury together at Sundance. A year later, Rick called me and told me about this script, and how he wanted to make a very low budget film that we can shoot it in six days and utilize miniDV. I was very interested in doing something very low tech. I got the script and it was so good, the actors he had were good and he is a good director. With that, I couldn't lose.

> I might even go into a store in South America and see this GRIM fluorescent light in the back, with a yellow light on the side and think, "Hey, that looks great. That's a good iDea."

## Had you worked with digital video before?

I worked with this tiny little video camera on [Michael Apted's] *Me and Isaac Newton* (1999), which I shot in mostly super 16 blown up to 35mm, but there I used it to give the piece texture, and to create more expressionistic images, not to tell the story. It did give me a taste of this little camera. It is tiring to keep a big camera on your shoulder all the time or in a car. You want to do traveling shots in Madagascar—we were crossing great landscapes and you don't want it always on the shoulder; I did some images where the side mirror is in the frame. One of the landscape, one in the mirror. You can do fun little things in that.

## Did you do a lot of tests?

No. We really didn't have a lot of time to do that. InDiGent, the producing company, in a way, tested it for us. Gary Winick, one of the partners, had directed a DV movie called *Sam the Man,* and Ethan had just directed a movie for them called *Chelsea Walls* in miniDV. They had shot they with a PAL Sony PD 100, and everyone at the time seemed to think that was the right camera. The camera was very small. It literally fit in the palm of my hand, and we could place it anywhere. That would be impossible, and/or time consuming with a regular 35mm, or even with a 16mm. It was very freeing for the actors and for myself.

## How did you approach the shots?

We built the motel room on the soundstage and then lit the room with a lot of practicals and removed a part of the ceiling. Rick divided the script in five parts, and the actors had rehearsed a lot, so they really knew the story and their lines and would go through script ten minutes at a time, and we would do four or five passes over those ten minutes, but nothing was really planned as far as blocking.

## Did Rick shoot as well?

I was the A camera, the main frame, he was B camera, meaning I had the best spot and he had to squeeze in and fish for the little things. He is so great; I joked with him, "Is it the air in Texas that makes you so mellow?" He is a very strong director, but very much a collaborator. What I really tried to doing during the passes was get new angles or the same ones if I thought they were very strong. And I think in this way, *Tape* gives you frames you don't normally see in movies. And there was this flow of ideas that was not interrupted by the sometimes cumbersome technique of filmmaking. I felt very free. If I had an idea I felt instinctively I could move there. Frames were not planned, they would come into my head and I could go and do it in two seconds, and you don't have that on a film. Three people alone in a room for an hour and half...it could've been quite sterile. But the film has a lot of energy because nobody was stopped by the process of filming. There was no resetting or fussing with lighting; we just went and for me it was great because I felt I was part of the performance in a way. I was right there, very close to the actors, so it was also a lot of improvisation for myself as well. I think because the tools were so small my imagination was a lot freer, all at once, and it keeps going and the frames keep on flowing. On *Crumb*, I nearly fell off the roof, which would've have been a lot more critical, but here, if I wanted to jump on a chair and shoot above the lamp, or go in someone's armpit or press myself against the wall and have a pane of the wall in the frame, jump around and climb on the bed or the couch I could do it all. I really feel what we lost in terms of image clarity we gained in terms of the excitement of the visual energy of the piece because of DV.

**Looking at the film, it seems that the actors enjoyed it just as much as you did.**

For an actor, it is like a dream come true. You can go ten minutes or for more and there is no cut and reset and go back to your trailer. It's pure performance.

**What problems come up working this way?**

I haven't seen enough movies in video, but for the few I've seen I think that a lot of the mistakes that people are making have to do with the fact that they want to make it look like a film. I think, especially with the little cameras, it's never going to look like film, and if you are trying to go that way, you are shooting yourself in the foot. It is not film, but something else, and that should be understood and exploited. One of the problems now is that everyone is a director; the actors, the producer—everyone wants a shot at directing. It's the new glamour in the art world.

But you really need to know what to do. You can have a great crew, and all the great tools, but if you don't have the director you don't have anyone leading the troops. The director is the central artist of the piece, and if that person is not there, the piece is being made by the soldiers. There is center, no core. I am one of the main artists, yes, but I am going to do my best within the best structure. Not when the directorial work is put on me and on everyone else.

**DV can be excellent in documentary work. You can catch things very quickly due to the invisibility of the camera. In retrospect, is DV something you would have used in shooting *Crumb*?**

I can be invisible with a 16mm camera! But no, *Crumb* has a look that I think is great. I don't think every documentary should be shot in video. And I don't think, "Hail DV, celluloid is dead." Video has its benefits, because it is inexpensive and you can just shoot everything. Again the problem can be that you think, "Oh, I can make sense of all this footage later," but that's not true. How and why and what you shoot still all has to make sense. After *Tape* I was approached by a lot of people who want to do movies in miniDV. They send me the script, thinking just because its in miniDV, it's going be done in two weeks. That isn't understanding the medium. Shooting on video does not negate the art of makeup or costume or lighting. We still have to light as carefully as one does a film, unless you're shooting a Dogme film.

the problems NOW is that everyone is a director; the actors, the producer— EVERYONE wants a shot at directing. It's the new GLAMOUR in the art world.

**Why do people think this way?**

People are so used to TV as being reality. It's an art form that crosses every race, every class. We are so used to that type of image. We call it reality, but the technical aspect of the frame, the grain of celluloid film is closer to what the eye sees than the line of the video.

**Did working on *Tape* make you appreciate the more reflective experience of a 35mm feature?**

Reflective? Honestly, on a bigger film, there are more things to deal with, in regard to the pressure of the politics, the money, the producers and all that. On films like *Happiness* and *Velvet Goldmine*, there wasn't a lot of reflective time. There was not enough time, not enough money, and they are both very complicated movies. For only $5 million or $6 million. The time for reflection is in pre-production, when you are still working in the abstract. On the set for movies like these, which are so ambitious, the problem becomes keeping your vision within the bigger machine.

**Do you plan to shoot in DV again?**

Of course. It's here and it's a tool and if something comes along that I feel is a good project, I'll do it. The great thing about it is once you've shot, you can go back on the Spirit or the Renaissance [machines used for film to tape transfer] and you can fine tune your film—adding contrast, isolating color, really playing with the image. It's used a lot on music videos which are shot on film. They used it on *O Brother Where Art Thou?*, which was shot on 35mm. They went to tape to give it that look and then went back to film. There are so many different possibilities.

**And what's beyond DV then?**

I don't know…maybe implants in your head? The future is wide open.

## ( JOHN BAILEY )

John Bailey, ASC, first entered the world of cinematography via the graduate program at the School of Cinema/Television at the University of Southern California. Following what was then the traditional path, Bailey joined the camera guild, and spent eleven years apprenticing as a crewmember with such notable DPs as Néstor Almendros, ASC; Vilmos Zsigmond, ASC; and Don Peterman, ASC.

Since 1978, Bailey has compiled an eclectic body of work, with over forty feature films including *Ordinary People, American Gigolo, The Pope of Greenwich Village, Racing With the Moon; Mishima: A Life in Four Chapters; Silverado, The Big Chill, Brighton Beach Memoirs, The Accidental Tourist, In the Line of Fire, As Good As It Gets, Living Out Loud, The-Out-of-Towners* and *Divine Secrets of the Ya-Ya Sisterhood*. As a director, his filmography includes *Via Dolorosa* and *The Search for Signs of Intelligent Life in the Universe*.

*The Anniversary Party*, starring and co-directed by Jennifer Jason Leigh and Alan

Cumming, is the first film Bailey has captured on digital videotape. Even so, he says he views the film as more of a hybrid between the two, as it is a movie made by traditional filmmakers using the tools and techniques of this newer medium. Following this aesthetic, *The Anniversary Party* was printed and exhibited on film.

**You are well known for shooting big 35mm features. What interested you about working on *The Anniversary Party*?**

Over the years I have done smaller projects. I am hoping that one of the things that will happen is that I will get approached and offered more unusual, edgy things. I like doing a mix. I've done documentaries all along. *Via Dolorosa*, which I think is an important statement on one of the most defining political crises of the last fifty years, I shot on super 16. But insofar as *The Anniversary Party*, as I recall Jennifer was very keen to have my wife [editor Carol Littleton] and I work together on the project. I suspect that it has something to with the kinship Carol and I feel to an earlier film we worked on together, *The Big Chill*, in that there's a central reunion and that it basically takes place in a house over a very compressed period of time where a lot of friendships are thrown into question.

**You shot on the European Pal 25 frame system, which promises a clearer, more resolved image than the American NTSC. What cameras did you use?**

A Sony DSR500. We tested two other cameras: the Canon XL1, which is a wonderful camera, and the Sony PD150, which at the time was a new version of the PD100 that a lot of the Dogme films used. We shot in PAL because everything we had been led to believe was that we would get a significantly better quality. Which we did. Twenty-five frames is much more filmic. We finally decided on a DSR500, although it's a much bigger camera and weighs almost as much as a Panaflex, because it has a 16x9

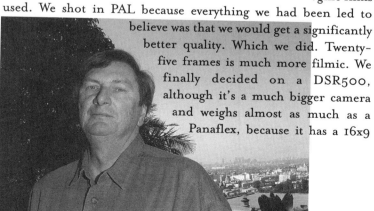

DP John Bailey.
photo by Larry Hammerness

chip and therefore it had a lot more information capture than the others would have had.

We used the DSR500, for the most part as film camera, on a dolly with controlled compositions; the film isn't shot in the Dogme style. There are several sequences in it that are shot handheld and with very little light and there are certain sequences that were shot just with existing light. And there is a crucial scene, the climatic scene, that takes place away from the house, while Sally and Joe are looking for their dog and have a huge fight, and the marriage breaks in half during the course of the scene—that was shot with very, very little light. We tried just using a lantern, but everything was just black, except for the lights of the city, and it looked too phony. I used one supplemental light, just to define the ground, the path they were taking in the bushes, but it has a real Dogme feel to it. It was shot pretty much handheld, very rough, very much like Lars von Trier's operating style, but it was really right for the scene. Because even though Jennifer and Alan are very disciplined actors, this was a raw and brutal spontaneous scene. It was totally scripted, but we wanted the sense that everything is falling apart, so I shot it as much as I could in the Dogme style.

**How did you discuss the shoot?**

I was surprised at how visual both of them were. Jennifer had been working for a long time in preparation while Alan was shooting a film, and Alan came in very close to the shoot. Jennifer had been doing a lot of thinking about it and Alan made storyboards, which are not conventional story boards—they are renderings he did of some of the key sequences, kind of like cartoons or drawings. They were very helpful for the two of them together to think about how the scenes should work.

**This was the first time you've worked with DV—were you nervous?**

I wasn't nervous at all. I knew exactly what was going onto the monitor was going onto the tape. It was easy. It is very easy to light for video, because you don't have to make any kind of extrapolation about how the fill light, or the kicker or the balance with the exterior is going to work. You'd see the dailies. One thing that is terrifying but also very magical about film is that it's an inexact science. It's analog, it's unpredictable. You don't always know what you're going to see and things sometimes turn out differently than how you think. As a cinematographer I have shot over forty films, so shooting on digital video was kind of a walk in the park. Technically, things like balancing to the exterior were a lot more challenging and the video chip doesn't let me have the latitude, but what I saw on the monitors and on the wave form gave me a very clear idea of what we were laying down. It's like looking at your negative as you're exposing it.

**Did you miss the unpredictability of celluloid?**

I actually prefer the surprise of celluloid. I would go look at dailies the next day, and there would be no surprises. The other thing is, and a number of directors have spoken of this, when you are shooting on film and sitting next to the camera [as opposed to a monitor], like a lot of the older directors still do, no matter how aware they are of what they think they're getting, when go they go to see dailies—blown up, sitting there in the dark room, totally lost in the experience with nothing to distract them—they are always surprised. When they see with what is happening with the actors, the subtlety and the unpredictability is always a revelation.

> You don't know what you have until the end when you RENDER it to film.

With video you go to see your dailies and you're looking at a monitor, and it's pretty much the same size as the monitor you had on the set. In fact, a lot of times, you don't really see what you've gotten until you've edited the sequence and you take your Avid output and project in the theater, and even then, it's such low res. The fact of the matter, and one of the real liabilities of digital video cinema, is basically you can't see what you're movie looks like—and I'm not talking about the cinematography, I'm talking about the drama and the performance. You don't know what you have until the end when you render it to film. And by that time you've made all of your decisions in the editing room, you're pretty much locking the picture based on looking at low res images and for the most part looking at it on a small video monitor.

**Do you feel that this approach has altered the content?**

I think there's something very different that happens. For me, as an analogy, I think the style of editing movies—film—changed drastically and quickly, when the Avid started to replaced flatbeds. And everyone says, "Well that's MTV and commercials and the influence of the cutting and the pacing," maybe so, but bigger and more tragically, it's the easy, quick manipulation of a nonlinear video editing system. You can push the buttons, you can rearrange, you can make the cuts so quickly, and people get used to looking over and over at a small screen, so everything gets cut into close-up and extreme close-up. You hardly see movies anymore that have an establishing or master shot that lasts more than four or five seconds.

For me, it was one of the big problems I had with *AntiTrust*. When I went to do the digital mastering, the telecine for the high def master, every cut is labeled an event, it's a number of cuts. There were almost 2,000 events, or cuts, in *AntiTrust*, which is by far the largest of any film I've ever done. I'm used to dramatic films that have 700 or 800 cuts in them and this was more than doubled. Now admittedly this was a quick-cut, contemporary action film, but unfortunately, that's becoming more and more the rule. Even character-driven dramatic films are being edited so fast.

**Agnes Varda said that what she missed working on DV was the reflective time she experienced while cutting celluloid. That it had more of a sense of creation and that influenced the making of the film itself...**

Technology influences style, style influences content. Carol started on a Moviola, then she went to a flatbed and then she went to an Avid; she says that one of the thing she misses most about working with 35mm film is having it in her hands and having to splice and thread it. While her hands were doing all the mechanical, busy work, her mind was thinking about the process. She said that that reflective time, when you are evaluating your work, considering things, even overnight, or playing back what you've done, is very crucial to establishing dramatic density. Now it happens so fast. Every producer, every studio executive, every actor in the film can have their own cut of the movie on an Avid. And you get into situations where you've barely presented the director's cut and then next week you got five different versions of the film for the execs...it's chaos.

I think it's being reflected in the kinds of films we're doing. Films are losing their center, their singular point of view. The filmmaker's point of view. Between that and the test screenings, focus groups and previews, everything is getting so sanitized and homogenized. The bar is being lowered. All these things—the drama, the complexity, the richness of characterizations and ambiguity even, which is inherent in any kind of poetic medium, is an anathema to guys like Joe Farrell who go around and conduct these preview screenings. "Oh you didn't understand that? We'll change it...." So films have become much more literal and audiences are being dumbed down—and the more audiences see dumb films the dumber they become.

### Do you feel that this generation of filmmakers possesses filmic literacy?

It's a very different thing, to have a foundation, literacy in terms of literature and culture that you can kind of break off from. Young filmmakers today are cinematically literate but they don't read. They haven't read a Chekov short story, and so they don't understand the basics of construction, or narrative.

You look at the French New Wave and you look at all the great innovators, whether it's Godard, Rohmer, Truffaut, Malle, Rivette—they were incredibly literate men in terms of the classical French tradition of reading. Truffaut, we know from *The 400 Blows*, had a very messed up childhood but read even as a youth. There's that wonderful sequence where "Antoin Doneil" builds that little shrine to Balzac. And, even though he and Godard were knocking down the old fashioned barriers of film style, they had a tremendous reverence for the literate text, and you see it especially in Truffaut as he went deeper and deeper into his career, where by the '70s, films like *Adele H.* are almost literary films.

### Younger filmmakers seem dazzled by the possibilities opened up by Dogme 95. Yet von Trier and Vinterberg, for instance, had made films on celluloid before they moved on to DV. Do you feel this experience assisted them when they began to play with DV?

Absolutely. I was on a "Film Is Dead" panel at Sundance last year—I've had a tremendous sense of living the past year with this kind of hectoring, argumentative position that people have taken. Either film is dead or video is crap. But they are two different mediums. While they can reinforce each other and they can interweave, they not only coexist but they can interact creatively and amicably and that's what they should be doing. For instance, I would love to do another video film, but that doesn't mean I'm going to give up celluloid. And the fact that I've done a video film doesn't mean that I've done it and seen it and am no longer interested. There is no reason not to continue to do both.

**In *Traffic*, Steven Soderbergh seemed to interweave the two ethos.**

A lot of *Traffic* was done in such a way where you could feel that it had a newsreel quality to it. It was a very interesting choice and it is one of the things that gives the film the tension and the drama that it has. It is a very scattered and diffuse film in a lot of ways, but the cross-cutting of different stories, telling them in an immediate, you-are-there way, acts essentially as a unifying element.

**Video is supposed to provide a more real representation of reality, but there is a flatness to it. Why does film feel more realistic?**

It has something to do with the nature of the way the images are captured. A film frame is unique—the structuring, the patterning, the grain in the individual frame is distinct from another frame, so each frame is completely refreshed, and it has a different quality than a video image. A video image is captured on a chip that has pixels, and the pixels don't move. The metaphor I use is that it's like an image on a group of mosaic tiles. This image is different because there's something about the grain and the analog constantly shifting quality of film celluloid. It has this dream-like quality, it's smooth and embracing. There's something haunting about it, it's not literal. If you take a video image and render it to film and put film grain into it, it will have a filmish look to it, but it's still not the same.

The worst thing of all in terms of looking artificial, is this hyper-realistic, artificial look when you have video capture and a video projection or transmission. That's the worst, and I think very few of the people arguing for digital projection in the multiplex—which would be the first phase of this transformation—are arguing to abandon film capture.

**If photography freed up art, is DV freeing
up film?**

As far as I'm concerned, we're right at the infancy of whatever
the interface is going to be, because digital technology is still so
new, still so primitive in a way. From the point of view of students, it really empowers them. They can go off with no crew and
virtually no equipment, even if they aren't producing anything
of a very high quality. If they have something to say, if they have
ideas and energies that they want to get recorded, they can do it
very easily.

From the other end of the spectrum, you have people in the
studio, in the marketing, distribution and exhibition end, who
really want to get rid of film because it is so expensive and bulky.
If you're doing 2,000 or 3,000 prints of a film, you're spending millions of dollars—$1,500 a print—each of which then has
to be shipped. If they have either a direct transmission or some
kind of Internet cable transmission, it's a lot cheaper.

**Then why does one get the impression that the
studios are not so keen to move over to digital
projection? Or to validate DV films as real
cinema?**

I do think they are interested in having DV film for distribution
and exhibition, but very few of them have been done in such a
way that would appeal to a mass audience and the studios, let's
face it, are not interested in the art house movement. *Chuck & Buck*
aside, the money for them is if they can open 1,500 to 3,000
screens on a weekend. So I don't think that the technology is
good enough yet to capture images of high enough quality to satisfy the audiences that go see these huge event movies. Now Lucas
thinks that it is, and he's betting his reputation in a way on this
with the newest *Star Wars*.

**Lucas is shooting the new *Star Wars: Episode II*
on 24P HD. Because of its higher definition,
he says that the results are indistinguishable
from film.**

Many filmmakers are convinced that celluloid film is still far
superior to digital videotape in all regards—tone, texture, color
and the capacity to resolve detail and complex patterns. There
are also lots of skeptics in the special effects industry who have
done lots of tests with that camera. People over at Disney—in

their so-called Secret Lab—have done stuff at higher resolution than Lucas has available on this camera. What we have to realize is that the Sony camera he used, that he's going around saying is indistinguishable from film (and all of us who have looked at it know better), is essentially a one K resolution. It's 1080, just over a thousand lines, and anything that is being done at the minimum CGI effect on a film-to-digital element is being done at a 2K resolution and preferably at a 4K resolution.

There are a lot of people [Joerg Agin, president of the Entertainment Imaging division of Eastman Kodak] who say, in theory, if you were to scan a single frame of 35-millimeter color negative film—and depending whether you use a whole frame like anamorphic or you have a 1:85 extraction—you could convert it to a digital file of 9 million to 12 million pixels and you could essentially get at least a 6K, 8K or 10K image, depending on how much of the negative you used. The amount of information in the detail is significantly different. In pixel count the CCD recording chip of a Sony HD camera is basically 2M pixels.

**And as far as the digital projectors go?**

That's another thing. The equipment is changing very fast. We've had the JVD and the Texas Instruments DLP System, but both of them are being replaced because they've hardly ever been installed, because they're still in a testing phase. But there are several new and better generations of projectors coming out, and it's very possible—assuming the studios and the exhibitors can reach some kind of agreement on who is going to pay to put these in theaters—that we could see a lot of them going in.

**Who will take the first step?**

The marketing divisions of the major studios are pushing digital exhibition very very hard, because they can save an enormous amount of money. It's also about control of the image. For instance, if they send out a 35mm film print and an exhibitor who has a multiplex can shift it around, he can move it wherever he wants; he can even have unauthorized screenings. Once that print is out there, anything can happen because it's strictly an analog system and can be duplicated very easily. But digital projection will be controlled from a central place by the distributor. It can be encoded and every machine that projects that image will only be able to do it when it has the proper code to unlock it. Meaning, if I understand correctly, each showing on each projector will essentially be encoded and decoded by the distributor so they will know exactly when and where and how many times the film is shown. The studio will have complete and total control over the exhibition and showing of everything that they put out there—until of course, somebody breaks the code. The point is, the exhibitor will not be able, at his discretion, to start moving stuff around.

**That scenario sounds remarkably like Big Brother. But might not that still be to the good? Especially as film projectors by and large are not receiving upgrades commensurate with projection standards?**

Well, I'd be the first person to admit the projectors are in terrible shape and it is really a scandal that the exhibitors and distributors have not insisted on high upgrading of projection standards the way they have with sound and Dolby and so forth. They have not insisted upgrades for the picture quality, so picture quality can be very bad. It looks great at the DGA, but if you go back to the Midwest—to Oklahoma, where Carol's from—and walk into a multiplex in suburban Tulsa, God knows what you're going to see. And yes, there's a case to be made that at the bottom end things get very, very bad, but what nobody seems to be addressing is that the same kind of denigration and corruption of the media is happening with digital, too. When it happens in digital, the images break down completely. I have seen projections five or six times and I have never once seen it without some kind of breakup—and that is in controlled situations, in demonstrations where you have the engineers from the studio essentially supervising and maintaining the equipment. What's going to happen when they start selling these projectors to some guy with two theaters in a small town in Nebraska? This guy is going to hire someone who's not a video engineer to run it, essentially the same way he runs a film projector. And what about when the DV stuff starts falling apart? It seems to me that the amount of maintenance required by a DV projection system has got to be astronomical and far more labor intensive than it is for any kind of film projection system. This is something no one is really talking about.

> It seems to me that the amount of MAINTENANCE required by a DV projection system has got to be astronomical and far more LABOR INTENSIVE than it is for any kind of film projection system.

### So digital video exhibition is not as cut and dried as many of the proponents would have us believe?

In fact, the standards aren't even in place yet. Everybody is dealing with pie-in-the-sky about how we're going to get these digital projectors in and they're going to run great and look so great, but I was at a meeting of the advisory group which is trying to set standards and we got into a discussion about that whole issue because they're doing testing of pieces and comparing compression ratios and things like that. There is so much data that has to be transmitted along these lines, whether it's satellite transmission or some kind of Internet thing, and it all has to be compressed. And whenever you compress and decompress images, depending on how well it's done, there is a compromise of quality. And when you get a drop-out you get a real drop-out. When we took the video master to film on *The Anniversary Party,* we had several problems, unexpected glitches and things that had to be redone.

### So, although film stock is more expensive, the technology is more simple?

At the ASC clubhouse, we're gradually getting a lot of old equipment that was in storage; light meters, filters and personal memorabilia from the old cameramen. A lot of the old cameras—the old hand crank ones going back to 1910—are gradually being put into working order. We have an archivist who is a cinematographer, but he shoots a lot of music videos and he has used them in his work. You can take any camera that is 100 years old or more and if it's in mechanical order you can put in stock, shoot, send it to the lab and there is a film image. Whether it was photographed in 2003 or 1901, it's a real image. And they're all compatible and will run in any projector in the world.

### What about the shelf life of video?

DV is new. Videotape is not. Videotape came out in the mid-50s, and we started having all these formats that changed during the '70s and '80s. The formats were changing so much. We discovered that videotapes essentially had a shelf life, or a half life, and the material would start degrade in ten years and have to be upgraded to a new format. The thing is, the formats themselves are disappearing and the machines that recorded them and can play them back are obsolete. There have been over seventy video formats developed since the mid-50s, all of which are basically incompatible and all of which have to have their own machines to record and play back. We are losing a lot of information—for instance, NASA has lost tremendous amount of information from the Gemini and Moon programs because the machines just don't exist anymore. Terry Sanders did a wonderful documentary about the loss of information on the video medium, but essentially they have had to go back and rebuild machines that have been junked, and bring people out of retirement who were engineers and who knew how the tracks were laid down.

**There is also disintegration with these miniDV camera heads, isn't there?**

They are magnetic heads just like the ones on your VCR. After a while, you do have to replace the heads. With film cameras, such as Arriflex and Panavision, if you rent them from a camera house, you know how they have been maintained; the technology is called mature technology, which means a whole system of standards have already existed for generations. This whole DV thing is so new and there are so few standards and so many neophytes involved and the equipment is all so incompatible—God knows. It's a crapshoot when you go out with this equipment.

**If money wasn't an object, should students be trained on more old fashioned equipment and then move on to DV?**

That's a hot point, but it's also comparable with the speed of our overall culture. How many college students read the original Flaubert, or even the Cliff's Notes? It's endemic and pervasive in the society. The pace of everything now is that we want instant empowerment, instant gratification. As I am not a film teacher, my personal plan would be to start students on video so they can see how easy it is to capture images, to give them a sense of comfort and empowerment and satisfaction. So they can actually go out and do something and then go look at film equipment. Then I would teach them the principles of filmmaking using film equipment and let them decide what medium they would want to use.

But I think the problem is that several years ago an overnight change took place. When I was in film school in the '60s, all we had was film, but by the '70s and '80s, a lot of students were doing their first year projects on video—and they hated it and they couldn't wait to shoot 16mm or 35mm. Now that's changed.

All they want to do is shoot video, they start and they don't want to give it up. They don't want to be bothered to learn all the nonsense about film because to them, film is a dead medium, it's not going to be around. Why should they learn about exposure and how to light and so forth if they've gotten so used to the automatic tools of video?

**Did you enjoy working in DV on *The Anniversary Party*?**

Yes, it was a lot easier in a way. But I never felt I had the creative palette or the subtlety. It is much more elemental. It's not bad, and was certainly appropriate for this film, but I was very aware of it and had to change my lighting style completely. There was a learning curve for me, but that's one of the reasons I wanted to do it. But because I could see the result immediately on the monitor and I didn't have to wait the next day to see dailies, I could determine very quickly that I couldn't light in this way, or this has too much back light, I need more contrast, and so forth.

That instant gratification one gets with video, which has it's down side, worked in an interesting way for you on the upside....

*They don't want to be bothered to learn all the NONSENSE about film because to them, film is a dead medium, it's not going to be around.*

It was very exciting, there was truly as sense of immediate construction. You really felt in doing it that you were in fact making the film. That what you were capturing was exactly what you had—and especially on our schedule, which was just nineteen days—to achieve a two hour film of theatrical quality was exciting.

**Did you shoot a lot of tape?**

Not that much footage. There is a charades section of the film in which they all do performance pieces that were somewhat impro- vised. We used three cameras for that. Most of the film was shot with one camera, sometimes with two.

I would say DV is good for people who think they want to use video because they are going to shoot an enormous amount of stuff—it is so much cheaper. But with *The Anniversary Party*, we were making a fairly controlled, more traditional film. It is a hybrid, as it is shot on video in a film style. We also did very few takes, with many of the scenes done in only two takes. I still think that if I would've shot it on film, I could've done it seventeen days because film doesn't require the constant maintaining, balancing, white balancing of leveling. There were a lot of things that slowed me down and, to me, they were at least as time consuming as anything that would happen on film.

**The Anniversary Party tells the story of an intimate gathering of friends. With the superfast shooting schedule and with such a high-profile Hollywood cast—Kevin Kline, Phoebe Cates, John C. Reilly, Gwyneth Paltrow—was there still that increased intimacy everyone always talks about in utilizing DV?**

I think for the actors there certainly was. We referred to it as a home movie, because there is something about the environment that is created by shooting on this sort of videotape. The camera we used was a larger camera, but all the actors felt that there wasn't as much at stake, so they were kind of loose and free.

I know there are arguments to be made on the other side—the pressure you are put under when you have a camera running at ninety feet a minute and you only have a limited amount of film, so you can't screw around. When the director says "action" you better be there. If you know you can do twenty or thirty takes on video and one can only do two or three on film because of your budget, that is a significant factor in the time that it takes to make a movie. I find, personally, it's not the set up or lighting time, but the amount of time it takes to do take after take. Maybe you spend forty-five minutes lighting something and two hours shooting it. In any case, you can make an argument for both ways. A lot of actors like the rush, the focus of energy and tension that they get when the film camera runs and they know there's a lot at stake. It galvanizes them. Some feel intimidated and threatened by it and the thing they like about video is that it is so casual and throw away.

**Some actors feel they look like crap in DV movies.**

Well, that's true enough.

**You grew up viewing filmmakers such as Scorsese, Coppola, Friedkin, Schrader and De Palma, all of whom fell under the spell of the French New Wave. Why is Godard being referenced more and more in the last few years?**

Even at the time, Godard was a great metaphysician—he was the intellectual and theoretician of the New Wave. Not only did he write about the polemics and the issues of investigating and interpreting the medium of film, that ethos itself exists in his movies. In his early movies, his characters talk about movies—they talk about the movie that they're making in the movie. There are touches of this self-reflexivity in Truffaut, but nothing like Godard. He is the most self referential of all filmmakers. At a certain point after *La Chinoise* [1976], he abandoned film and started making video, and became more and more experimental. He went back to film eventually but there was a whole period, the Maoist period, where he was strictly into the politics of the medium and I mean that not just in terms of Maoist politics, but in the philosophy of image capture.

**He has been a huge influence on filmmakers.**

Certainly, because of style and content—he blurs the two so much in a lot of his early films. This evolving style was essentially part of the content of the film. I mean, it's hard to think as far back as *Breathless* [1961] with the emotional and the dramatic momentum being separated from the way it was shot and edited. In *Le Mepris* [*Contempt,*1963], the opening shot of Raoul Coutard is the shot of the cameraman on the BNC Camera and it comes rolling toward on the dolly track in profile and at the end it turns toward you, the audience, and tilts down so that the lens is focused right at you. The French New wave filmmakers, certainly at the beginning, saw film as a weapon, as an aggressive social political tool. The energy in the early New Wave was an energy of aggression, not in terms of violence like it was in America, but in its emotional and ideological assertions.

**Do artistic restrictions and political divisiveness bring out the art and idealism in filmmakers?**

My own opinion is pessimistic. My view is that things are going from bad to worse to the degree that all media is being controlled by larger and larger more consolidated conglomerates. And that is the degree to which the content is going to be homogenized

They say, "Here's your CAMERA
and your set and you capture
and it goes into an Avid or a
G4 PowerBook and boom! boom!
Make your movie and boom!
Right to the Internet, no studio
executives, no development,
no previews, no BLA BLA BLA."
It just doesn't work that way.

and rendered harmless. I think we have less and less edginess, roughness, experimentation. We will always have independent and experimental films, and certainly Sundance has given a lot of creative forms tremendous exposure. But the studios, the content providers—they own publishing houses, which can decide what books get published and that will be strictly on the worth, on it's power to sell versus what will expand to challenge the medium of literature. It will depend on how these ancillary markets can be exploited.

So many publishers are now part of the information and communication conglomerate, or creating their own. Even if the maverick and independents continue to make their own work— and everyone talks about the Internet as a great medium that's going to expand everything—but the studios are getting into the Internet. And as soon as the system is up, the conglomerates will be exploiting it. They will respond very quickly to the technology. So, even if people can create alternative content, how are they going to get it shown?

I've seen these flow charts that trumpet the great thing about DV. They say, "Here's your camera and your set and you capture and it goes into an Avid or a G4 PowerBook and boom! boom! Make your movie and boom! Right to the Internet, no studio executives, no development, no previews, no bla bla bla." It just doesn't work that way. The middlemen who can control it will get in. It's the inherent nature of the way things are and that's human nature. I've been inside this system for a long time and see how this stuff in fact actually happens. And the total freedom some are expecting, well, that is pie-in-the-sky.

## ( ANTHONY DOD MANTLE )

Cinematographer Anthony Dod Mantle, a long and lanky forty-five-year-old, doesn't so much arrive in a room as materialize in a mercurial burst, as if determined to engage as many particles of energy as possible.

And this may also be the way he works. His electricity brings forth the mad, the poetic and the ideological in all of his eclectic collaborators, who include film-

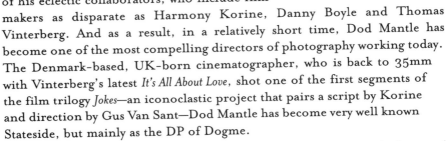

makers as disparate as Harmony Korine, Danny Boyle and Thomas Vinterberg. And as a result, in a relatively short time, Dod Mantle has become one of the most compelling directors of photography working today. The Denmark-based, UK-born cinematographer, who is back to 35mm with Vinterberg's latest *It's All About Love*, shot one of the first segments of the film trilogy *Jokes*—an iconoclastic project that pairs a script by Korine and direction by Gus Van Sant—Dod Mantle has become very well known Stateside, but mainly as the DP of Dogme.

This notoriety stems from the fact that Dod Mantle has lensed three of the six "official" films shot under Dogme 95. The films include Harmony Korine's *julien donkey-boy* (for which Dod Mantle was nominated for a Spirit Award); the Berlin Film Fest winner *Mifune*, directed by Søren Kragh-Jacobsen; and the Cannes-winning family drama *The Celebration*, written and directed by Thomas Vinterberg.

Viewed within this frame, it may seem as if Dod Mantle is the DP King of Dogme, but he rebuts gently, "I want to be very clear about this straightaway. First of all, I've had a very short career. I've done lots of commercials, a few documentaries, but I've only shot eleven features, and only three of them have been on DV. Secondly, Dogme doesn't have anything necessarily to do with digital filmmaking; it's about the process, it's about naked storytelling."

"But oddly enough," he adds wryly, "these bloody Dogme films have drawn more attention to me as a DP than anything else I've ever done. It's partly hype, but perhaps it's because in these kinds of films, the cinematographer's work becomes incredibly visible. There you are, hung out for the count and there's no coming back."

Dod Mantle, who grew up in the South of England, arrived in Denmark for the first time in 1979. "I had lived in London for five years, and had become a still photographer," he notes. "Got involved with Denmark, via a woman of course. Went over there for a while and after the relationship fell apart, I thought, 'Why the hell have I been learning this language?' There had to be a predestined reason. I refused, because I'm so stubborn, to get on the next plane back, and instead applied for the National Film School [the school Lars von Trier and Vinterberg had also attended] and got in on my first try."

It's not merely the country, nor the "convenience" of working with such talented people that inspires him, says Dod Mantle. "Whenever I do any kind of project, I have a gut feeling that can be adjusted or developed. And this happens organically. For *Celebration,* I was witnessing a story of a family decomposing, slowly disintegrating and I decided I wanted to find an aesthetic that could bring it out. With Søren's film, which is tighter and more classic in approach, he and I were in total agreement from the beginning that it was a celluloid story."

And with Korine, Dod Mantle invented a banquet of tricky spy cameras to emulate the grainy, inner realm of a character's schizophrenia. "Visualizing that from many different points of view seemed to be the right way to go," he says.

Dogme, he offers, is definitely provocative, as it insists on a reduced technical palette as a more challenging way to create. "But that is a benefit and for me, not an end in itself. I can't trigger my fantasy until I've sensed the soul of the project. That happens early on, when I see the script and begin to visualize what's between those lines. Whether it's a Dogme film or a conventional film on digital or celluloid, I begin in a terrain of space which is inspired by a story, which is initially filled by myself and the director and the scriptwriter and actors. That's where the magic begins."

As for his increasingly high profile, Dod Mantle laughs, you will encounter his favorite claim to fame should you click on his Web site. As the opening page rolls into view, you'll hear a surprising audio clip excerpted from von Trier's *Breaking the Waves.* "Anthony Dod Mantle," a patriarch's voice thunders over an image of a windswept grave where several religious elders of the secluded Scottish village look on, "you are a sinner and you deserve your place in Hell!" If you click onto the next image, you will hear the voice of Emily Watson's character Bess echo agreeably, "Anthony will go to Hell, everyone knows that...."

Says Dod Mantle modestly, still rather pleased with the tweak, "It's kind of a homage, I think. Due to scheduling and other things, Lars couldn't find a way to use me on that film, so he found this way instead. And I have to say, I don't mind at all. But next time," he deadpans, "I'll just have to demand more time in front of the camera."

## Dogme has become very much associated with digital video, hasn't it?

Yes. And I want to be very clear about this straight away: Dogme is not about video; it is about the organic process. The intimate collaboration between a director and DP is an organic and private process that gradually unfolds itself. It is difficult to control. You have rules. And the Dogme rules, as Lars says, are just rules. There could've been only five rules or twenty other rules. The fact is we always have rules no matter how sophisticated the film production, and we happen to have these ten rules but they could've been other ones. Whether a Dogme film or a conventional film, I begin with the story; there is a space, and the space is inspired by a story and initially filled by myself and the director and the scriptwriter and actors. Already there you have a kind of frame, an apparent limit to a territory of thought. That's where you begin to create your ideas. That's where I begin to find a way that I can visualize another person's thoughts.

To be quite honest, Dogme is provocative because my palette is smaller. I find certain weapons or utilities taken away from me. But the process is the same. You have some rules, you work within those rules, and that creates a certain freedom. I welcomed this concept with open arms, because it was playful. And, ironically enough, as a cinematographer, for some strange reason, there has been a larger focus on me as filmmaker because of these three films. In my short career so far, I spent fourteen years committed to celluloid, the gamma curve and the beauty of sophisticated lighting and controlled mood. And suddenly, with the Dogme films there has been an immense focus on my craft as a cinematographer. I don't know what that's about, but it's interesting.

*Ewen Bremner in* julien donkey-boy. photo by Anthony Dod Mantle

**How does Dogme alter your relationship with the director?**

My experience in Dogme has polarized the increased intimacy of the working relationship. Søren would be sitting next to me whispering in my ear, "Anthony, I don't think I can see my actors any more. Can you? Can the camera? Can the lens?" If I'm working within a normal set-up on a film and I have my lights and my wonderful crew and all my beautiful technical people to help, the director will take for granted that the DP will take the time they need. But with this way of shooting, there is preparation, but you don't have that delay.

**Lars von Trier shot almost 80 percent of *The Idiots* himself. Do you think he should have had a DP on that project?**

Lars was shooting *The Idiots* at roughly the same time I was shooting *The Celebration* with Thomas, and in the early days we talked a great deal about how it was going. He found it exhausting holding the camera up like that, but beyond that, I understand Lars well enough to know now why he shot *The Idiots* himself and why he was quite content to do that. He was in a phase where he was denouncing—to a certain extent—the concept of framing, the concept of a metaphysic with in the frame, and I don't agree.

**You didn't follow the Dogme rules to the letter in *The Celebration*.**

I've commented on the cheats I made in *Celebration*—putting the camera on the sound pole, which is hilarious, and it's also been documented in the film. You can see the reflection in the mirror. It's a little macguffin. But the rules could've been "Stand on your head, close your eyes and film." People are focusing so much on these rules—it's absurd! Obviously there is an element of precision, but the concept is about a larger canvas, to make you think.

**On *Celebration*, what was a typical day during the shooting of like?**

They'd all come in, sometimes sixteen people, and we'd stage to a certain extent the small things with the main actor. I actually didn't block it as much as I normally do. I'd run the entire tape through because I promised myself I would never stand in the same place twice, except to cover the speeches. I had multiple cameras covering the reactions and fear of the extras. But because of this concept I had of moving out of control myself sometimes—I am on my feet so I need some kind of control—I was free to do the takes all the way through without cutting.

**You seem to have so much of your spirit invested in _Celebration_.**

Werner Herzog talks about finding truth through creative stylization and fabrication, and I think there is a combination of movement and space and time and incredible technology in the film. The thing is, I've seen the film so many times and that it's a part of my body and soul, and as a result I have great difficulty seeing it objectively. The reactions are extraordinary on many technical and spiritual levels, so in answer to you, for me as a cinematographer, I think, touching on the essence of mastering the craft—the science, the artistry—I hope that out of all this technical, scientific process comes truth. I think about it every day.

**In working on three of the six initial Dogme films, how did you manage to keep a fresh point of view?**

One can still be quite spontaneous. The only reason I did three is because they were sufficiently different from one another. And making a Dogme film doesn't mean wobbly-wobbly running around. It lets the process be free, lets the actors have space and it lets us be spontaneous in ways to shoot. Thomas was full of playfulness and Søren is the only one where it could've been shot classically. But he let me go and let me what do I wanted to do.

Harmony was exploratory, as you know he can be and which he has been criticized for, but I like him for that. Using all those spy cameras, hidden cameras, looking for one-off exchanges with people on the streets. In dealing with a man who is schizophrenic, intuitively it seemed a logical recipe to use different angles and observe from different viewpoints. As soon as I would approach Harmony about having a more structured recipes, as DPs like to do, he always said, "Just do it from the gut." It was really a privilege to work with someone like that.

**What was it like going from DV in _Celebration_ to shooting _Mifune_ on celluloid to _Easter_ back on DV?**

For _Celebration_ I wanted an agility that wasn't possible with a film camera. I have had many conversations with my colleagues around the world and I could've shot on Panavision, I could've had a thousand ways to do it, it's a very traditional narrative, very tight. But I had no intention of pushing *Celebration* anywhere near an image that I had seen before. I shot it the way I did because I wanted to disappear as much as possible into the group of people using the smallest cameras. I wanted to make movies that were more emotional and out of control. Less intellectual. Of course, I used any possible molecule of intellect to create that kind of workspace for myself.

But once I made that decision and created that technique, I wanted to be invisible to people. I wanted a small camera at the end of my arm moving without my intellect. I was witness to a story of a family's slow disintegration and I decided I wanted to find an aesthetic that would could bring it that out...and I found this odd grainy organic mishmash that ended up as this massive screen image in Cannes. It was extraordinary to see this image that was so far from anything I had done before. And I don't sug-

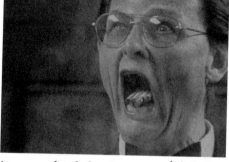

gest that it has any aseptic quality I can respect or disrespect, it was just the look I wanted.

When it came to *Mifune*, as it is very expensive to shoot a lot of film, we had to be more in control of the process—we also had to move the speed of the film to give access to darker spaces to be exposed correctly—which is part of the reason we ended up shooting one third the footage than the other Dogme films. It was a lovely challenge. But whenever I do any kind of project I have gut feeling in my body of what kind of approach I want to take, what kind of format I want to work with.

*The Smoking Man in julien donkey-boy.*
photo by Anthony Dod Mantle

When I did *Easter* with Gus Van Sant I would have to say, I was forced into making it a digital movie. As an imagemaker, it was initially against my gut feeling. But I could sense his feelings as a director were strong enough, and he was teaching me something so I went with him on it...and now I think we did the right thing.

But insofar as working within Dogme, it's like a playpen...you let the child play, but you put a bloody wall around them—you know, let them play as far as the road. There's always a limit, and a frame is just a line around a frame. Like I said, something is always going on outside the frame. You can't dismiss metaphysics.

### How many hours of footage did you end up with on each film?

For *The Idiots* I think Lars came home with 160 hours, on *Celebration* I think it was eighty-eight. And on *Mifune* we came home with twenty-three hours.

### In such a collaborative atmosphere, where does the ego come into play?

I have actually been very annoyed with some of the press critics dealing with Vinterberg's camera and von Trier's camera. It's abysmal. There is this fetish about the director not being credited and there's obviously been an incredible cult of personality. I'm the one saying all this, but it's not coming from insecurity. If you want to be a DP, you have to accept the fact that you are, to some extent, a mystical figure behind the camera and that's okay, it's part of the Karma. It's very different, very difficult being a director and getting the slaps in the face all the time. But there are some fundamentally idiotic tendencies in the press. It's the cult of the directors, the cult of the stars, and it's not informative or educational for the cinema public. Yes, at the end of the day, it's a collaboration. I'm so grateful to my assistants and my production designer and my light crew. Obviously they're carrying energy through the process and it's a long haul for them. But it can also hurt. It is a delicate, sensitive, very little talked about world between directors and DPs. It's a very sensitive area....

> But insofar as working within DOGME, it's like a play-pen...you let the child play, but you put a bloody WALL around them—you know, let them PLAY as far as the road.

### And as for your relationship with von Trier?

I met him fifteen or sixteen years ago and kind of danced around him. He teases and plays sometimes at being a recluse and I'm so glad he hasn't become a Howard Hughes with long hair and long fingernails. When I met him the first time he had finished the script for *Element of Crime*, his first feature. And I came back to Denmark and watched it on the editing table as it was becoming the film it became. I was meant to shoot the first *Kingdom* and I couldn't—I was shooting a film in Mexico—and that was the beginning of a very strange relationship between us where journalists thought there was something weird going on because I said "no" to Lars. Honestly, I was just tied up. I shot elements of [the Stig Bjorkman documentary] *Transformer.* I shot Lars' first wife's [Cæcilia Holbek Trier] feature. It was documentary on opera singers which Lars' company produced, then she got money for her first narrative feature which is about nuns which was all shot in a studio [*Nonnebørn* (1997)]. I shot films that his company Zentropa has produced, as well as shooting the dance sequences on *Dancer.*

**Dancer in the Dark's dance sequences were extraordinary. You used an anamorphic lens— what did that do?**

You put a special lens in front of the camera and you get a 16x9 format which squeezes the maximum amount of information to the new format so you don't lose pixels or resolution. It's kind of annoying and semi-consuming because you have to screw something on and it can slip out of place and get twisted. It's not easy to work with.

**Who would you choose if you were to choose a DP?**

It wouldn't be Lars, I'll tell you that. I'd have that man tied down with sixty rules.

# Beyond Dogme

**Mike Figgis**  united kingdom
RISKING THE FUTURE

The joy of the Digital Revolution is that one can use a camera the way in which one uses a word processor. In a way, it's what Godard had always asked for—please make me a 35mm camera that I can put in my glove compartment. He also always said, quite sagely, that filmmakers should own their own cameras. That's never been possible unless you are a very indulgent or very successful filmmaker and even then, the size of the equipment would be daunting. With this new technology, I'm really thinking of situations now where I will just be with my actors by myself, with no one else there. And how wonderful that might be. I've always been a stickler for that, always owned my own 16mm equipment and continue to and I have three video cameras: a DS500, new digital widescreen, quite stunning, and a DS100 DVcam which is also an amazing camera, probably the most interesting because it's tiny...all three chips...all PAL. I'm about to buy a night vision camera—that has to be really interesting—all of which can be used in various film-

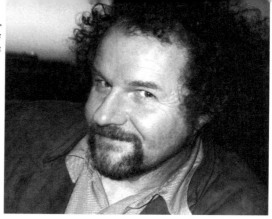

making situations, and I have an Aaton super-16, which is time coded, so it's the latest in film technology.

Sure, DV makes filmmaking more available to everyone, but everyone's got the availability to write a bad novel, too, and that didn't destroy literature. That's the problem with the marriage between literature and film—so much time is spent talking about film. It also means what Steven Soderbergh said, that there'll be many more bad films available, but of course, by definition there will also be more potentially good films being made—and made in the context of a non-studio environment, which as far as I'm concerned can only be wonderful, really, because I think that a studio is the least creative environment for filmmakers that one can conceive of. And one of the currents of modern cinema is that it's this world language of Hollywood stories. It fills me with horror. There is of course, a real deep-rooted resentment of American product all over Europe. I think it has something to do with what Ingmar Bergman said...he could never work in America or anywhere hot because his brain didn't function.

I haven't shot on 35mm since One Night Stand. I love it that people compliment me on my celluloid films, which are all shot on super-16.... Leaving Las Vegas and Miss Julie and The Loss of Sexual Innocence were all super-16 films. If you use a much slower standard stock the blow up to 35mm is so good here in Europe that even film people can't tell the difference.

But as far as this new 24P HD camera goes, I have no interest in that whatsoever. I'm not interested in clinical reproduction, which seems to be offered by the 24P HD camera, I don't think I really ever had been. "Oh boy, you get a

flicker option that makes it look like 35mm...Oh joy!" Grow up! To me that is the worst kind of fanaticism. Not only are 24P HD cameras extremely expensive—and so bloody sharp apparently that you've got to buy a completely new set of lenses that doubles the cost of the camera—and then you think, "Hang on...you're competing with 35mm which is already pretty good in terms of image recording, and this is like an impersonation of something which already impersonates the way we look at things in the first place." The new generation of low-end digital cameras are really quite stunning.

So, in regards to all the divisive dialogue of film vs. DV, I think people always overreact at the outset of any new technology.

I think it's our nature, I think it makes us insecure when new things pops up. People clung to Steenbecks and flatbeds, insisting that it was somehow closer to the spirit of cinema, when all that had happened was that someone invented a better system. Avid and Lightworks and all that—it means many things. If you are looking at something like five times more films being put onto the market, clearly that would create a saturation beyond what already exists. So you come up with alternative theories of distribution systems, and in that case there's more room for the esoteric and there's more room for different and diverse kinds of film and so on.

To understand what is going on in the digital revolution, it's probably instructive to look at the performance-art movement of the last fifteen or twenty years to see what they've done, what kind of explorations they've made since they discovered video. I love that video looks different, I love the kind of arty quality of it all.

I do still view cinema as an art form. I wouldn't want to have anything to do with it if I didn't think that.... I also think it is the most oversubscribed whore in the art world now. But that doesn't mean it can't regenerate and be a pure form once again.

I shot TimeCode on DV and transferred to celluloid for theatrical release, and yeah, it put a huge whack on the budget. It also reinforced the silliness of it. It's times like that when you realize what a dinosaur the Hollywood film business is because of its inability to move quickly and come up with the goods, because their capital investments are so vast in stuff they've invented, which is the stuff designed to make even more money each time. Maybe they've overinvested to the point where they've become incapable of moving quickly, which is just a wonderful opportunity to come out with something else. When those things happen, it's rather good for filmmakers because you almost get an open market. Right now, the minute you sign on to any sort of any Hollywood thing, you can forget the love bit in a way because by definition you will have given up much of the freedom you had on your first film and then the hardest thing becomes to express yourself some way which isn't just a compromise.

It can be like when you make your first record; you are Fiona Apple or Massive Attack or whatever, everybody wants that sound, wants some of it. Everyone says, "Wow the next album is going to be astounding!"

Of course, the second or third of anything means you're in the business of having to deliver and that's really tough. You now have entered the business of being a filmmaker and that's great and you want to keep on doing films because it's a good job. It then becomes—unless you're Kubrick or someone—something where you have to produce the goods on a regular basis. But there's no spontaneity to that and now you're not making it for the same reasons you made your first one.

Around the time of all the Hollywood hoopla of Leaving Las Vegas, it felt like high comedy. Highly enjoyable high comedy. If you had to do it fairly regularly I imagine it would be very dull, but as a one-off it's fantastic. Still, I was just as happy to get on and make another film. To be honest, I enjoy filmmaking far more than being lauded. You are always rendered so passive. When someone comes up to you and says, "I've just got to tell you, you are the greatest thing since sliced bread," there's not a lot you can say. You can't say, "I agree," you can't say, "Rubbish!" so you are rendered for quite a long time as person who can only find horribly

> I do still *View* cinema as an art form... I also think it is the most oversubscribed WHORE in the art world now. But that doesn't mean it can't REGENERATE and be a pure form once again.

English ways of saying, "That's so frightfully kind of you." The only option is one of movement, always seizing the opportunity and carry on making films as quickly as possible...practicing with the medium so that it becomes more of a natural voice, rather than a thing that one visits every couple of years for a special occasion. At the same time, I believe that if you are perceived as being arrogant it's not the end of the world. It's important to say those things sometimes and prepare to be counted for it.

I've sort of gone through my own Dogme, in a way. I made rules for myself, pre-Leaving Las Vegas, and I kept to them for the most part. They have to do with the ability to shoot a film in a certain way, at a certain speed, at a certain budget and make it story-driven while still giving the actors the kind of room where I might get great performances out of them and still retain control. Those are very practical survival rules for me, but they were formulated not in a not very formulaic way at all. It's all about having a story, although story is very negotiable; it's really about making a very strong film. Sometimes a strong piece of art. There can be no hard and fast rule about content. The only thing that really applies is, having seen it, it feels right, so you just know, don't you?

Certainly Dogme must take the credit in a way for legitimizing DV. I probably helped, being foreign. Certainly the American culture looks for endorsements and a standard of approval from a European source. Those Danes—those guys turned up out of nowhere as far as everyone was concerned—and clearly they had a terrific attitude and that certainly got through like a rock group to a whole generation of filmmakers. It's almost like the punk movement. The actual statement is as important as the films they made. The Dogme manifesto is laughable in a really good way. The big danger is when these things are taken terribly seriously and become religious dogmas and quite the opposite of what they were intended to be because people so need a religious cult. But like movements and like clubs, again the Hollywood club. So how can you keep on being risky? I would define risk as feeling as if you didn't have to join that club. Really the risk of being an individual, that very American thing which everyone treasures and prizes, but very few people take the option of and I think in the UK, God bless them, there's always been an element of individuality and pride. It is really a small country.

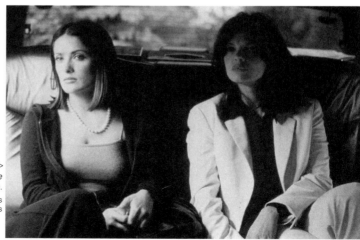

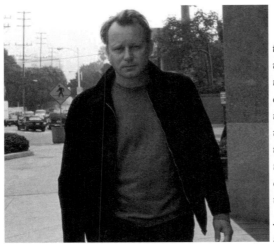

*Stellan Skarsgård in* TimeCode.
courtesy of Mike Figgis/Screen Gems
photo by Elliott Marks

Everyone realizes that the price of the technology will bring the price of projectors down. Seattle, Minnesota, it can be DYI, do it wherever you want...we're very close to the point where we don't need the studios...and I think they are starting to realize that and it's making them a little nervous. It's the sort of paranoia that the ten buckets of gold that you've made might be reduced to eight. They already make so much damn money in the cinema, I find it very hard to take any of their arguments seriously. They are just about greed, and what I love about the new technology is that it's like this rather clever child that sort of leapfrogs around the back of all this....

One of the fundamental things that will probably come out of all this is that, without a doubt, all cinemas will have to become digital. It is a much better idea than celluloid projection and one could have a far better product and we will further develop the video techniques, which are now accessible. It's a bigger menu, that's all. But given the economics of America and the economics of the film indus-

try...whatever innovation comes along will be massively exploited for its economic potential, first and foremost. If one can make cheaper films, it will increase your profit and more people will get ripped off in that way. But on the other hand, it also opens up the market and the potential for filmmakers who maybe want to work outside of that system.

Now, I'm working on kind of an extension of TimeCode, technically speaking, trying to go farther with those techniques. [Hotel, shot on location in Venice, Italy.] The joy for me at the moment is to be able to be risky, to move quickly and not have the next four years planned out.

There is a buccaneering, romantic aspect to making movies, and I think that's one of the more exciting things about it, really. The thing is, whatever the medium, I have found I don't look for perfection in camera or in performance. What I do love is when a certain energy is hit by an actor and one starts to see how extraordinary that person is, in that moment of creation. That's what I love about it all. That's why I want to make films.

The big *DANGER* is when these things are taken TERRIBLY seriously and become religious dogmas and quite the *opposite* of what they were intended to be because people so *Need* a RELIGIOUS cult.

# RIDING THE EDGE:

## DIRECTORS

With Lars von Trier's *Dancer in the Dark* becoming the first digitally shot film to win the Palme d'Or at Cannes 2000, digital cinema has achieved a massive victory. The changing terrain of the filmic medium, reflecting the strengths and transitions of Hollywood, European and independent filmmaking, calls to filmmakers who have worked in both celluloid and digital video. Turning to the new medium, they say, has helped them to explore innovative ideas, where their independent film spirit can reemerge.

Within this new collective; Alexandre Rockwell's *Thirteen Moons*, Hal Hartley's *Book of Life*, Mike Figgis' *TimeCode*, Allison Anders' *Things Behind the Sun*, The Polish Brothers' *Jackpot* [shot on 24P HD], Jonathan Nossiter's *Signs & Wonders*, Spike Lee's *Bamboozled*, Wayne Wang's *Center of the World*, Agnes Varda's *The Gleaner's and I* and Richard Linklater's DV double headers *Waking Life* and *Tape* join the growing roster of seasoned directors willing to take their spin behind the medium.

For most of them, it's not like they've given up on their love affair with celluloid. DV simply means less time spent cooling their heels between films, and more opportunity to risk experimental terrain. Given DV's smaller crews and lower budgets, there is no symposium of nervous, newly creative money-men to impose their voices on the material because they think they know what will sell. Once again, the director is free to tell a story. And if, even with this newfound freedom, the movie turns out to be less than picture perfect? As Samuel Beckett once said, "Next time, fail better." A mistake is often just an opportunity that has lost its place.

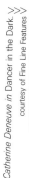
*Catherine Deneuve in Dancer in the Dark.*
courtesy of Fine Line Features >>

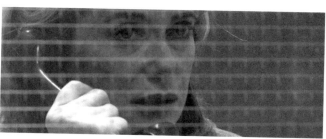

# ALLISON ANDERS

A deeply personal filmmaker who is unafraid to weave her private experiences into the fabric of her films, Allison Anders followed *Grace of My Heart* and *Sugar Town* with *Things Behind the Sun,* her third consecutive feature to deal with music industry lives. Carrying a bruising emotional kick, this deeply personal film also draws on Anders' early-adolescent trauma as it centers on two people damaged by a rape and their struggles to confront the past.

Anders, who grew up in rural Kentucky, was only five when her father abandoned the family. Raped at age twelve, she suffered abuse from a violent stepfather and by the age of fifteen had fled with her sisters and mother to Los Angeles, where she suffered a breakdown and lived on the edge of sanity, shuttling between mental wards, foster homes and jail. By twenty-two, she found herself a single mother, with two daughters by different fathers.

Enrolling in junior college and later the UCLA film school, she was completely taken with Wim Wenders' films, and so deluged the filmmaker with correspondence that he gave her a job as a production assistant on his 1984 film, *Paris, Texas.* Three years later, in collaboration with two of her classmates, she wrote and directed *Border Radio,* a headlong dive into the L.A. punk scene. She still struggled on welfare up until 1992, when she made her solo writing and directing debut with *Gas, Food, Lodging,* a trailer park saga about a mother whose two adolescent children are growing up too fast. Her evocative *Mi Vida Loca,* a gritty tale of girl gangs in her Echo Park neighborhood in Los Angeles, followed the next year.

In *Things Behind the Sun,* Anders wrote with her *Sugar Town* collaborator Kurt Voss, shooting for the first time on DV.

During post-production, Anders selectively enhanced the colors, particularly the harsh rape scenes, via computer. For the shooting itself, she purposely utilized a restrained, filmic approach involving smoother shots, and more classically composed framing than what is usually associated with the inherent freedom of digital video production.

**Why did you decide to shoot *Things Behind the Sun* digitally?**

Originally it was because it was cost-efficient, but now I'm so sold on the technology that it will always be a creative decision. I was really happy working in this medium, and especially happy doing the post in the film. And I love how it looks—it looks very different from film. Things went quicker, although maybe not that quickly, because a lot of the characters had to deal with putting in hair extensions. But seriously, if you don't know it's digital, you'll know there's something amazing about it but you won't know quite what it is. It has this unique quality you can't get on film.

**Did it change your approach to shooting?**

Yes and no. I didn't get gadgety at all. I treated this movie like film and composed it very carefully. It is in a wider screen than I usually shoot. I probably went for more composition and more careful lighting than I've ever done with film. I treated it every step of the way like film. The advantages are that even when you spend a lot of time lighting a scene, it still takes only half the time to set it up. You have more mobility with the camera, and more time with the actors in front of the camera.

**How much of the film is your own history?**

Not much. Everything in this film is fictionalized and everything is true, but there are some serious autobiographical elements about where the rape takes place. I went back to the town where this happened to me as a kid, but even so, it's not an autobiographical; it's a pretty fictional film.

**Did your approach to the sex scenes came from a more sensitive, female sensibility?**

I wouldn't have thought so, and now that I think about it, probably not, not from some of the stories I've heard. But for me it does come from a very female place, because I know that women's bodies have been very misused in cinema. I am probably more sensitive to actors—male actors as well. On *Mi Vida Loca,* we had to shoot a sex scene and one of the guys came to me and told me he was getting shit about it at home and we discussed it.

Male actors tell me what they won't tell a male director. This stuff happens all the time, but they will tell me about it. It's kind of burden because you still have to get the scene done, yet you have to be sensitive to the personal part. I totally went for it dur-

> *I think what often happens with SEX scenes DIRECT them. They kind of go, "Okay...do that stuff..." and leave the actors to their own devices. It's always nerve-Wracking.*

ing the shoot, but it required going over it every step of the way with the actors.

I think what often happens with sex scenes is that directors don't direct them. They kind of go, "Okay...do that stuff..." and leave the actors to their own devices. It's always nerve-wracking. I find it very scary to direct sex scenes. You always have to plan it out, and there's always anxiety about what's going to be shown, how you're going to cover up things. It's an ordeal.

**Still, it must have been interesting directing a sex scene with two brothers.**

Oh, the *menage á trois* scene with Kim Dickens, who plays Sherry the rock musician. In my twisted thinking, I thought an actor would be more at ease doing a sex scene with his brother, and they agreed with me. They felt that they could trust each other, and they would prefer it, because they felt they could really keep that boundary secure within the scene.

Basically your job as a director is to make the actors feel safe. That's it. So they can give performances, give you their feelings. And these aren't just sex scenes—they are sex scenes that reveal character and past trauma. Everything was very choreographed and rehearsed.

**Like musical beats?**

Music is really important in this movie. Not just because the characters work in music, but also because it's how they both deal with the pain in their lives. They use pop songs as an escape, as well as for inspiration.

**Do you have "Anderisms"?**

No, but there is a trust, especially with Eric Stoltz, whom I've worked with so much. I needed to be able to trust all of these actors in this movie because this film was so intimate, so personal for me. And I think using the DV also worked well in that way.

**I've heard that you were influenced to use DV by Dogme 95—is that true?**

I loved *The Celebration* enormously, but this film doesn't look like any of those films. I didn't move the camera a lot—there's a little handheld stuff, but it is really smooth. But before I began shooting *Things Behind the Sun,* I was toying with the idea of doing it in the Dogme 95 style. I even went to Copenhagen, to Lars von Trier's company base Zentropa [where he shot a lot of his *Dancer in the Dark*], to find out more about Dogme 95 and shooting digitally. But after thinking about it, I realized...the problem is, why would you choose to confine yourself to a bunch of arbitrary rules? I've already got that. It's called Hollywood.

## JENNIFER JASON LEIGH & ALAN CUMMING

"We are so well known for being actors," says Alan Cumming of fellow thespian Jennifer Jason Leigh, his directorial collaborator on *The Anniversary Party,* "that we were always very aware of the expectations. But one can't rely on other people's opinions. If you do, you'll become a nutcase; and now that our film is premiering in Cannes," he adds just loudly enough for everyone in this noisy West Village restaurant to hear, "we can just gloat."

A study of marriage, sexual distrust and promiscuity of the heart, Cumming and Leigh's DV-shot collaboration marks the feature directing debut of both in a story they also produced, wrote and star in. And while it doesn't push barriers with its portrayal of sex on screen or the woes of marital unrest, it casts a fascinating spell. From the opening scene where Leigh lays alongside her husband, gazing at his sleeping face with a combination of longing, pain and love, *The Anniversary Party* probes feelings with almost a blind person's sensitivity to touch. It's exhilarating to watch a film that searches emotionally for where it's headed, and unlike several current pretenders to the throne, it's truly an "adult entertainment."

Blurring fact and fiction the two portray Joe and Sally Therrian: He's a best-selling British author transitioning to film, she's an established actress undergoing a career crisis. Recently reconciled after a year's separation, a few affairs and recriminations galore, Joe has returned from London to the couple's Los Angeles home, where the newly cozy marrieds decide to celebrate their sixth wedding anniversary. Inviting their closest friends (who also happen to be Leigh and Cumming's real life friends, including Gwyneth Paltrow, Jane Adams, Kevin Kline, Parker Posey and John C. Reilly), Sally and Joe's "scenes from a marriage" unfold in one 24-hour period with a dreamy, bitter logic, and a deep undercurrent of mordant humor.

Since finishing *The Anniversary Party*, the art-imitates-life duo has been separated once again, this time by the reality of conflicting work schedules. The Scottish-born Cumming, renowned for his *Cabaret* turn on Broadway, and his eclectic character work in films as varied as *Titus, Josie and the Pussycats*, and *Spy Kids*, had a recently concluded return to the Great White Way starring in Noel Coward's *Design for Living*. Meanwhile, Leigh is shooting *American Beauty* director Sam Mendes' latest, *Road to Perdition* (a Prohibition-era crime drama based on Max Allen Collins' graphic novel that casts her opposite Tom Hanks), commuting between the Chicago film set and her native Los Angeles.

On a sunny afternoon at Hollywood's Chateau Marmont, Leigh sighs luxuriously and lights a cigarette, happy to be home again. "It's my one vice," she pleads, "but I really must give it up. When I go back to the set, I have to do an Irish jig, and smoking doesn't allow me much breath. You need your lungs to jig," she adds, exhaling a long, languorous plume of smoke. It is hard to tell where the smoker ends and the actor begins.

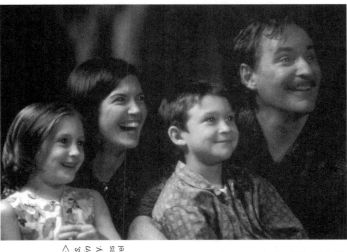

(l to r) Greta Kline, Phoebe Cates, Owen Kline and Kevin Kline in *The Anniversary Party*.
courtesy of Fine Line Features
photo by Peter Sorel

With nearly forty films to her credit, Leigh's portrayals of dark, wounded, tightly-wound women, fictive and factual, in films that include Uli Edel's *Last Exit to Brooklyn*, Barbet Schroeder's *Single White Female*, Lili Zanuck's *Rush*, Robert Altman's *Kansas City*, or Dorothy Parker in Alan Rudolph's *Mrs. Parker and the Vicious Circle*, have earned her a reputation as a quality actress willing to go to the very edge to find the heart of her character, a passion which served her well in her first foray behind the camera.

"It all began," Leigh notes, "when I saw the film *The Celebration*. I was doing *Cabaret* [also directed by Mendes] on Broadway with Alan. I went with my sister Mina [Badie, also in the film] and I was really floored by it. We were the only two in the audience laughing our asses off. But it was also totally shocking and horrifying, and so specific and so true, and of course, very inspirational. I was on the phone with my agent the next day. 'I must do a Dogme movie!'"

*The King Is Alive* followed in the summer of 1999, and Leigh was completely hooked. "I loved the whole process. It was amazing, the speed and the ease with which you can use DV—you could actually shoot a feature in three weeks if need be. After working with Kristian Levring on *King*, I wanted to make a movie, and I wanted to be able to make it within certain parameters: within the actors' schedules, and as inexpensively as possible, but with the kind of intimacy and immediacy you have with video. With DV I realized I could actually do it."

When Cumming visited L.A. last year they started talking about collaborating. "We decided that we wanted to do a story about a break up," Leigh begins, "and the way we wrote the script, everything was very specific, down to what needed to happen in every scene." Remembers Cumming: "The actual writing was very quick, but we spent months talking about the background, about the characters. With some of the cast, their friendships with Jennifer go back twenty years, so it was easy to write it for them because we always had their voices in our heads."

The fly in the ointment?

Cumming couldn't afford to give up his day jobs. Leigh continues: "We kept in touch by email and telephone. Sometimes it was hard to track him down because he was, literally, all over the place—Berlin, New York, England. I kept him apprised on the crew we were hiring, the actors we were getting, together with production office updates and how everything was going." She flashes an only slightly apologetic grin. "It was fine for me doing all that stuff, because—I admit it—I'm a total control freak."

"It's funny that I even made it to Los Angeles," says Cumming, who's busy displaying some his bruises incurred during pratfalls in *Design for Living*. "I'm a holograph in some of the scenes," he adds cheerfully. The actor, who has directed a couple of shorts (*Butter* with Helena Bonham Carter, and *Burn Your Phone* with *The Patriot*'s Jason Isaacs) had been toying with the idea of directing a feature, but adds, "I didn't feel committed enough to any project until this one. Initially, I was not a big fan of video. Ugly, ugly, ugly. You look like a dog. Which is why—although we shot it on DV—we didn't want it to look like that new crap aesthetic that people associate with the format. But, especially for this film, this story, perfect film would've been wrong as well. Here you have a beautiful life, but look closer and you see the fractures and pain." Leigh agrees." I didn't want jittery camerawork and bad lighting. I wanted the depth and beauty of film. Our amazing DP, John Bailey, really made that happen for us."

"Jen and I," says Cumming, "became like a married couple for a while. We'd order the same food at restaurants, we'd tell stories together at dinners, and during rehearsal people were laughing because we kept finishing each other's sentences. At one point we got a bit panicky, because we thought we wouldn't have enough money for post-production. So we considered getting married for a while, selling the photos to the highest bidder, then getting divorced right before the film was released." His dimples deepen. "It's a bit dramatic, but I still think it was a great idea."

### Why do people think you're New Yorkers?

*Jennifer*: Even though I was born and raised in California? Yeah, I love that. Because I wear dark clothes, I'm not dumb and don't have a tan.

*Alan*: Nobody thinks I'm a New Yorker. Okay, maybe it's because I'm very good with accents. I haven't used my own voice in a film yet. And yes, it's true, everyone from Scotland can do an amazing Sean Connery imitation. He is the king, after all.

### Were people surprised that you ended up directing a film?

*Jennifer*: Not at all. It was more of a what-took-you-so-long kind of thing. When I commit to a film, I have always been involved in pre-production. I do so much research.

*Alan:* I had directed two shorts before. People are always surprised by that for some reason. It's sometimes like Americans think that you didn't exist or do anything else before you came to America.

**Were there any surprises for you?**

*Alan:* I think actors in a pack are potentially quite a scary thing. They can lead each other on to bad behavior, mischief. You know what I'm talking about. The people in the film, even though some of them are famous actors, you forget that some of them need...reassurance. I had met them all, so it wasn't like a normal director-actor relationship where you've only met a couple of times. There was a level of comfort with all of them. Even so, I had to understand that as a director, I had a different relationship with each person. You have to understand what they need as people, and as actors to get them to feel comfortable and that can be tiring. You'd think I'd know this, being an actor, but when you are an actor too, and you're in the movie, it's quite bizarre. You feel a bit like a puppeteer.

*Jennifer:* For me it was fun actually. It's always fun to play the most harrowing, painful moments in life. The great thing was, in regards to my own self-neurosis, self-criticism, I didn't have time for it. It was a freeing experience for me in that regard. Because we wrote it, there was nothing Alan or I felt uncomfortable doing or saying. I think the speed that we had to work at worked in our favor. There wasn't a lot of reflective downtime, and what downtime there was, people were hanging out on the lawn, sleeping in the hammocks. A group of friends hanging out at the house.

**How did you balance at the directing chores?**

*Jennifer:* I feel shy if I'm in a party situation or a social situation where I don't know anyone. I also feel completely inarticulate in interviews, very self-critical. But I'm not shy when I work, there I have a place and purpose. If I have words, if I'm playing a part, it's easy. It's like taking flight. So producing a movie, editing, mixing, and all that—I'm very confident.

*Alan:* I think I said more on the set and Jen was more organized. When either one of us was acting the other was keeping an eye out.

*Jennifer:* We made a decision early on that we were not going to delegate to one another what tasks we were to do. We were going to embrace everything. We also agreed, if there was a disagreement, we would, take a "directors' moment" time out. But we didn't have very many. It was all pretty contained...we shot at the

house for nineteen days, which is a pretty short shoot. Some of
the cast worked only about two weeks, thirteen days or something. We didn't do it in a handheld Dogme format, we used
dollies, lighting....

### What was the size of your crew?

*Jennifer*: Sixty people, as opposed to 100 or 120 people. It was a
pretty big cast. Everyone had an hour to get ready and we had
three people who did hair and makeup who were really
great...but just to assist people, no one had one-on-ones. I
think we were budgeted at $ 3.6 million, which is probably a lot
for a digital film.

### What kind of camera did you use?

*Jennifer*: Our DP, John Bailey, used a Sony DSR 500 which is has
a larger chip and hence a larger camera as well. It's about the size
and the weight of 16mm, but because we weren't bringing in a lot
of equipment, we were allowed to shoot in this gorgeous Neutra
house which the couple wouldn't have let us into otherwise, and
shoot in canyons where it would be too difficult to get the equipment into. Obviously, with the larger chip camera, you can't get
into these tiny little corners—it didn't have the speedy compact-
ness that the some of the cameras, like the Sony PD150, has, but
the quality of the picture is much, much better.

*Alan*: We talked about how actor-friendly these cameras are. I
really like working in film, but there is always this kind of tension. "Okay, get to it, we got to get this get this now because this
is costing us *a lot of money* and we have *the camera rolling*!" It can be so
tense. With our film, it was all about people being relaxed with
each other. We got to forget the formality, and the "classic
order" of a film set.

### What format did you shoot in?

*Jennifer*: We shot on PAL, rather than NTSC, because otherwise
you are just losing so much quality. There are all these things
that are different and make the post process a lot longer and
slightly more complicated and tricky. With a DV movie, we really needed a good amount of time, in post, because there's a lot
of footage, so we had a full twelve weeks of editing [with film editor Carol Littleton]. Our mix was rather quick, which is tricky
with digital. You have to do pitch correction [vocals], which really worked, thank goodness. But when you transfer DV to film

everything slows down. PAL is 25 frames and film is 24 so suddenly everybody's talking so...much...slower....

### Where did you transfer to 35mm?

*Jennifer*: We tested everyone, we did these really elaborate tests.

*Alan*: We wanted it to look incredibly beautiful. For it to be rich, and deep.

*Jennifer*: And we tried all these different film houses, but we did blind tests because I was very prejudiced toward Hocus Bogus [where Lars von Trier transferred *The Idiots*]. I was a total snob for them, and I do think they are amazing, but in this blind test that we did, EFILM, which is in Hollywood, ended up being great. It had nothing to do with them being in town, or cheaper; everyone is very competitive in terms of prices.

*Alan*: I must say again, our film looks really beautiful. If you didn't know it was shot on video, you wouldn't even be able to tell. Yes, DV can be an aesthetic, can be a style, but we weren't going for that. That wasn't the point we wanted to make. We wanted to use digital video in a way that hadn't been done before. To make it a little more filmic. To push boundaries in filmmaking. That's what taking a risk is all about.

*Jennifer*: There are still a lot of limitations with DV. I have to say, the thing about video that really bothers me is the artifacting that you get, and the lack of depth a lot of times, because video is very clear, sharp. If you slow the frame, well you run into other problems. Warmth and depth, the way your eye perceives something is still very much the way film sees things and captures light. Video doesn't do that.

### Will you direct again?

*Jennifer*: Definitely. We'll probably each do the next one on our own and then maybe do another together again. But to make films that are very personal to you is so important. Even in acting choices I make things I want to see. Unless I really need the money, I try to make things I actually care about that are inspiring or challenging.

**"I'm fascinated** by DV. I think what's brilliant about the medium is that it really opens it up for young filmmakers. Independent film is generally an audition for the studios, quite often, but it will enable a whole new slew of young artists to do their own thing. And to me, it will mean with the money I have, I can do twice what I could've done on film. If DV can give me the quality that film can give me, I will use it in a heartbeat."

**TIM ROTH** / Actor, *Planet of the Apes*, director, *The War Zone*

And in order to make something that is honest and true, which also surprises you as well, the only way to do it is by just getting there.

*Alan*: I agree. But the next one is definitely going to be on film.

## MIGUEL ARTETA

Since debuting with 1997's *Star Maps*, Miguel Arteta has been keeping pretty busy. He's directed episodes of *Homicide: Life on the Street*, *Freaks and Geeks* and a pilot for Martin Scorsese called *Elizabeth Street*. And his newest project, scripted by Mike White, *The Good Girl*, starring Jennifer Aniston, might well be his bridge into the major leagues. However, it's his sophomore feature, the DV-lensed *Chuck & Buck*, which has given him the most pleasure. Influenced by the intimate revelations of Vinterberg's *Celebration*, Arteta's skewed look at "family" relations won't spur you to laugh out loud, but you will find a uneasy recognition rippling through your body as the film reveals more and more of the uncomfortable, compromising moments in life.

Produced by Blow Up Pictures (Open City's digital arm), *Chuck & Buck*, which debuted at Sundance 2000, is a wildly original and deeply disturbing tale of Buck O'Brien (Mike White, who also wrote the script) who exists in a state of suspended childhood, a twenty-seven year-old man who still thinks and behaves like an eleven-year-old. His childhood friend, Chuck (Chris Weitz), is now Charlie, a smooth record company executive who has grown up and thoroughly embraced adulthood, fiancée and all. When Buck initially tries to reconnect (with a furtive grope and a meaningful look), Charlie makes it emphatically clear that he doesn't share Buck's longing for the good old days, and continually (and unsuccessfully) tries to give him the brush-off. Undeterred, the consistently starry-eyed Buck obsessively stalks his childhood friend, moving to Los Angeles to stake out Charlie's workplace and home. Knowing no homoerotic boundaries, he uses every trick in the book to regain the love he once had, and the past he clearly refuses to forget. Sidestepping all stereotypes, Buck is no menacing marauder, but rather a lonely little boy wearing an adult's skin, and he desperately wants his old buddy to play with him again.

**"As long as** there is one laboratory on earth that manufactures film, I'll shoot on film."
**STEVEN SPIELBERG /**
Writer/director/producer, *The Sugarland Express, Saving Private Ryan, A.I.*

The visual aesthetic and style only increases the corrosively funny apprehension and underlying tension. Grainy, blown-out images enhance awkward events and memories, while the hand-held camerawork by Chuy Chavez (*Star Maps*), gives the film a fidgety intimacy that calls forth both empathy and repulsion.

**This is a pretty chancy movie. What are your influences?**

I love movies that are like good books where you don't want to guess what's on the next page but instead want it to be a real page-turner. I love the movies of Pedro Almodovar, of Todd Solondz; movies that make you deal with really intense emotion. Humor is the key, especially when the situations are extreme.

**How did you first start making movies?**

I went to every film school in the world. I went to Harvard University to make documentary films, but dropped out and ended up making fiction films at Wesleyan. Then I went to the AFI and thought I was learning how to deal with Hollywood. Then I realized that they weren't inviting me in, so I went out and made *Star Maps*.

**Where did you find the script for *Chuck & Buck*?**

From Mike White. I first met him at Wesleyan and thereafter cast him in *Star Maps*. He's now become a big TV writer, for shows like *Dawson's Creek* and *Freaks and Geeks*. I think *Chuck & Buck* was his reaction against the restraints of television. It's a very intense, twisted story. The two main characters are designed almost like the split parts of one person's personality. It's also a lot more raw in regard to human sexual relationships. Relationships are irrational and hard to understand. If it were simple, we would never fall into the trap of doing bad things.

**When did you decide to shoot on DV?**

After seeing Thomas Vinterberg's *The Celebration*. When I was thinking about it, I spoke to a lot people who had been involved in DV, in productions like Hal Harley's *Book of Life*, Harmony Korine's *julien donkey-boy*. People were very generous with information. At the end of day, I wanted the focus to be on the performances, on the story, and I felt this was the way to go. It gives you more possibilities in the way you can make the image look, and it gives an immediacy to the whole thing. I think for independent films it's great.

## How long was the shoot?

We shot for twenty-three days, and then did three days of reshoots. The digital thing wasn't a financial choice. We shot *Star Maps* for less money on 35mm. Using DV was a creative choice. I like the look of the video-to-film transfer. It has an intimate feel, and to be able to shoot with two cameras—I think they were both Sony VX 1000's—and to be able to shoot a lot of footage was terrific.

## What's the best advice you've ever gotten?

From Jonathan Demme. He really knows how to balance extreme situations with humor. That's one of the reasons why I always watch his movies before I direct. When I was his PA on *Cousin Bobby*, he said to me, "Directing is about responding, not about controlling." It was terrific advice that I've never forgotten.

## PETER GREENAWAY

The Welsh-born, English-reared, avowed post-Brechtian, deeply rationalist writer/director/painter/visualist, Peter Greenaway, sixty, currently resides in Amsterdam where he has lived for the past thirty years, ever since he met Dutch film producer Kees Kasander in the late '70s. "When I met him at the Rotterdam film festival," says Greenaway, "he offered me virtually a contract of a lifetime. He said, 'Do whatever you want, providing you're sensible and don't want fourteen pink elephants on an aircraft carrier, and I will support you financially.' It's been like that ever since."

He may not have directed the actual animals, but since 1966 he has concocted the hallucinatory equivalent. Dashing between far-flung locales such as Bologna, Paris, New York, Munich and Malmo to actualize his aesthetic aspirations, Greenaway is the intellectual's penultimate Renaissance Man. Obsessed by alternate ways of constructing a story outside classic storytelling structures, he is passionately fetishistic about utilizing scientific and natural systems such as number counts, equations and color coding to structure his ideas. He also approaches notions of sensuality with an extraordinarily vigorous and visual intellectual lust.

"An obsession with sexuality is the prime curiosity of the human race. It's those stretch marks between the notion of emotional identification and excitement, and also that very slightly stepping back that I am interested in. But that," he says amusedly, his uppercrust inflection an unmistakable point of view, "is very English as well."

Dangerously prolific and seemingly tireless, Greenaway has created art installations and one-man shows, written books, invented operas and of course directed a wealth of deeply original, outlandishly droll short and feature length films, including *The Baby of Macon; The Cook, the Thief, His Wife & Her Lover; Belly of an Architect, Prospero's Books, The Pillow Book* and *8 1/2 Women.* A formidable creative arc for a former painter who used to work as a film editor at London's Central Office of Information in the mid '60s.

In his career, notes Greenaway, he has unexpectedly received "an extraordinary amount of negative press in certain parts of the world. But I suppose I'm going to have to live with that. I'm certainly not going to cut the cloth to make a cinema that is easily acceptable. In some sense, it must be a measure of success to be the subject of such vitriolic criticism."

More and more, he muses, there has been a gradual tightening, and a remove from anything that might be considered to be experimental or

sensitive subject matter. "I remember what [visual arts critic] Susan Sontag said of [my film] *Prospero's Books,* a Shakespearean textural journey starring John Gielgud which marries and multi-layers the blatantly arcane and the excessively erotic. "She said," begins Greenaway, rolling the comment like an acrid plum, "Sontag said, 'it was a film of his visual indigestion. Mr. Greenaway is a cultural omnivore who eats with his mouth open.'" It was witty, if disparaging. But I make no apology about the huge amounts of visual information and I suspect I have fulfilled my ambition to create a work that needs to be seen an infinite number of times. We attribute those characteristics to poetry and music, why can't we do that also in film?"

The multi-contextual master is currently wrangling with a massive new project, *The Tulse Luper Trilogy,* which Greenaway has said that Madonna and Debbie Harry are to star in. It's an extravagantly conceived, three-part, six-hour film that he also plans to have digitally transmitted via the Internet.

Greenaway's launch into the brave new technological world may seem a shock to those accustomed to his "old school," lushly visual values. Even so, posits Greenaway, whatever the medium, "For me, what is shocking is really in the mind. My films are comedies in a sense, in a way that Ben Jonson might have used the word. They are deeply black and highly sardonic, as they are bizarre examinations of the most peculiar human conditions. Unfortunately, among certain audiences, I'm afraid I am taken far too seriously."

## Why do you think that your work still causes such divisive opinions?

I don't want to make comfortable cinema. All good art needs to be provocative. It certainly shouldn't be there to massage prejudice and underline what you already know. And I think the degrees of sensuality in a post-feminist sort of male reactionary world are something very interesting to contemplate and explore. It is quite terrifying really. All over the world now amongst the cultures, there has been a gradual tightening of belts and a removal of anything that is too sensitive. I've spoken to many curators in Europe and there is this great fear of a good Democratic society producing one member who can close down an exhibition because of the sheer process of a low common denominator, to have a vote and that vote becomes so powerful it somehow destroys the opportunity for everybody else to create a confrontation with culture.

For instance, I wanted to do an exhibition in Malmo, in Southern Sweden. I wanted five or six people to pose in the nude, which was an imagining of the future of the Olympics Games. Yet there is a very small Muslim community there and I was told not to do this because Muslim women are not allowed to look at naked men. I think to go out of your way to placate all minorities is quite disastrous.

But after 2000 years of Christ, it is very difficult to toss off all the traces and grains of particular attitudes. My particular position is one of neutrality. I'm not interested in closures and certainly not interest in the success of goodness, which primarily is the way in which most cinema is organized. Set up a situation of evil and find some solution for that. I'm not a political filmmaker—my interest has far more to do the with the aesthetic—but aesthetics is close to ethics and ethics is a branch of politics, so there you go. It's all interrelated.

## How did you end up in Amsterdam?

I discovered it was cheaper to make films here. Gradually my reputation grew in Europe, specifically in Holland, in Rotterdam, where I began to receive all kind of curatorial positions in the mid-80s. Then I became associated with the opera house and began creating works on a regular basis. One of them was recently at New York's Lincoln Center. It was called *Writing to Vermeer*. It's an appreciation of the extraordinary painting of Vermeer, who is one of my favorite artists. There is something very photographic about his vision. He has worked in the Netherlands in the 1670s. Godard suggested he was the first cinematographer because he dealt with the world entirely manufactured by light in split seconds of time, that Godardian notion that cinema is truth 24 frames a second.

In any case, I have found moving away from the silver screen to an operatic stage very freeing. There is a whole area of what is permissible, from notions of narrative and illusionism and reality, which I find very attractive. It gives me a lot of space in which to breathe. Werner Herzog almost exclusively does opera now. It might be the case that there is a license to attempt things on the opera stages that one is never allowed, or conventionally allowed, in the cinema.

### Why were you drawn to Fellini in your last film?

Fellini is actually not on top of my list of cinematic heroes. I would move towards Godard or Renais—who, for me, are the most cinematically intelligent moviemakers we have seen perhaps in the past fifty or sixty years. Fellini represents a visual tradition in a world of cinema that has basically become illustrated text and not the manufacture of images. He was also very influential for me due to his baroque nature. I'm passionately fond of Italy—I spent a certain part of my youth in Rome—so all that background is very familiar. I also admire his grammar and syntax, especially at the end of his career when he could always be extraordinarily imaginative in a direct visual sense. I think he also represents for me the apogee of European narrative filmmaking. I am basically anti-narrative, anti-illusion and anti-realism. So that makes me a rather strange cinematic product. But I think Fellini stands in a certain cinematic position that is really the beginning and end of cinema.

### You also take a great deal of pleasure in deconstructing many of those narrative elements.

Which is why Fellini is a dangerous influence in some way. But my cinema is very self-reflexive and that, of course, would appeal to me. Obviously I am initially fascinated by finding all the ways of constructing a film without using narrative. I do become excited about constructs. One can take from 20th Century paintings, number counts, equations, color coding and so and on and in that way find alternate ways to structure a film. But I make no apology about the huge visual amounts of information. With *The Pillow Book*, it was stripped down when it came down to text with image. The complications were of a different nature, but I think *Prospero's Books*, which was about an ancient Shakespearean text, had one building on something that had inherent archaisms, obscurities which I needed to make manifest, and *The Pillow Book* is obviously a contemporary tale.

One of the big criticisms and irritations people have about my cinema is that I am entertained, fascinated and excited by the form as much as by the content. I think that's because I was trained as a painter and I am still deeply interested in what the 20th Century has done to notions of vision and nonfigurative work. These are deeply problematical areas for most cinema-goers, who are used to going to view figuration, to see a tale, be patted on the head, and go to bed. So the provocations are always going to be problematic.

The idea of INDUCING the loss of control— the whole notion is SURREALISTIC.... Not for me; but the Scandinavians are PRONE to manifestos.

Of course, this is a cerebral construct, and if you show the skeleton, as I do, I think one should never deny other notions of the pleasure principle and my cinema is very much indeed about the world and its colors. It also shows a concern for the sheer sensuous physicality of what surrounds us. That is all very much part of the vocabulary.

**You did change the playing field for yourself in some regard.**

True. I set myself three problems. For *8 1/2 Women*, I wanted to make a film that had a great concern for a close-up, basically because my films are very much about wide shots. I wanted to make a film which had no music. Again, my association with music is considered to be part of my imprimatur, so I wanted to go against that particular characteristic. I wanted to return to the eloquent delights of excessive dialogue. To go back to the typically English wordplay of innuendo and conundrums. I haven't really visited that territory since *The Draughtsman's Contract* (1982) and that was a long time ago. In some way, this is almost a farewell to a certain kind of cinematic orthodoxy that I will probably not revisit again. I want to pick up on the possibilities that the new visual languages are offering us. And with *Tulse Looper*, I want to make the kind of James Joyce *Ulysses* kind of work which does make a true engagement of that potential.

## Rules against yourself...that sounds a bit like Dogme 95.

Yes, it does. I think one probably can understand why it rose, if only in order to fight the huge post-production now character-istic of American cinema, which doesn't just exist in America, but in Beijing, Turkey, all over the world. The emotions of Dogme 95 have been part of British cinema for ages. People like Ken Loach and Mike Leigh were making Dogme films before these people were out of nappies. To continue with the baby metaphor—it is like throwing the baby out with the bath water. You are foreclosing a huge vocabulary which is valuable. The Manifesto says there can be no post-production, certainly no music that exists off the set, nothing not generated by the actors, etc. Dogme becomes dogmatic. Manifestos are a terrifying way of ending up; they end up freezing you to death. The idea of inducing the loss of control—the whole notion is surrealistic. What did De Maupassant say? "The unlikely meeting of a sewing machine and an umbrella on a dissecting table." Not for me; but the Scandinavians are prone to manifestos. They had Kierkegaard, after all. In the paper once Ingmar Bergman was quoted as saying that he had long nurtured the idea of suicide. I find that peculiar, but then again he is a Swede. Making pro-nouncements.

## What films do you think are provocative?

The same issues, the same formalism, the same ideas go around and around and each generation never picks it up from the last. That's why I don't go to cinema. I find it boring to go as a social event. The actual event of going to the cinema and being stimu-lated for me is so rare. I do go to many painting exhibitions, I'm an avid reader, and photography interests me. Cinema is really a brain-dead pastime for me.

The last film I would've admired would be David Lynch's *Blue Velvet*, and that would've been a terribly long time ago. All the interesting radical people have moved on. Scorsese is still mak-ing the same films Griffith made. Underground cinema always stayed underground. Underground painting—like Picasso's—always comes overground, but underground filmmaking just circulates beneath the ice. Very few people actually get through and it doesn't become popular commerce in any sense.

[Luis Buñuel's] *Un Chien Andalou* and [Lynch's] *Eraserhead* are the few examples that have burst through.

**What do you think of your work after the fact? Do your films give you any excitement?**

You always wish they were better. I supposed I pursue the films something like eighteen months after I make them, mainly because I'm still proselytizing and travelling with them. But it's very rare to sit down and look at a film in its entirety and enjoy anything that I've made more than five years ago. I did see *The Draughtsman's Contract* in Hamburg not long ago, and it surprised me, but I hadn't seen it for about ten years. I felt as if it had been made by a stranger. And that must be good.

*Peter Sarsgaard and Molly Parker in Center of the World.*
*courtesy of Artisan Entertainment Inc.*

"**For** *Center of the World*, the thing that Wayne Wang came to us with in the beginning was that he wanted to make a film on video that looked like a porno, not so much in context, but in visual aesthetic. So he used lots of different digital cameras, bigger Betas, miniDVs. I think I kind of look like crap on video, but that being said, I think that he got some very interesting images. ❖ I think shooting scenes that are physically intimate is probably some of the hardest acting work to do. It can often feel incredibly fake and disconnected. Working digitally didn't necessarily make that easier. Yes, it was a fairly small crew and lights. But Michael Winterbottom's *Wonderland*, which wasn't shot on DV, had a much smaller crew and no lights. But the thing with DV is that after a while you don't notice it, or where it is. It's so small. It's not like when you're shooting with a 35mm camera. So sometimes we'd get to the end of the scenes and I wouldn't know where the camera was anymore and that can be quite disconcerting if you are trying to control some kind of image of yourself."

**MOLLY PARKER** / Actress, *Center of the World, Kissed*

# JIM JARMUSCH

Fusing his love of poetry and American pop culture to filmic sources as myriad as Carl Dreyer, Robert Bresson, the Marx Brothers and B-movie treats like *The Attack of Crab Island*, Jim Jarmusch films evoke a *Twilight Zone* universe somewhere near the crossroads of K-Mart and Flaubert.

On the map since Wim Wenders gave the up-and-comer the extra film stock to expand his thirty-minute short film *New World* into the 1984 feature *Stranger Than Paradise* (which subsequently won the Camera d'Or at Cannes), Jarmusch's wayward cultural travelers and enterprising foreigners have continued to stumble through worlds they will never fully comprehend. His strangers in strange lands include Roberto Begnini's Robert Frost spouting character in 1986's *Down by Law*, Johnny Depp's William Blake in the elegiac *Dead Man*, and the quixotic, Chaucer-inspired Cannes-winner *Mystery Train*. Even in *Ghost Dog—Way of the Samurai*, starring Forest Whitaker as a Monk-like assassin, Jarmusch seems to be dreaming of a greater beyond, some unknown course to be charted.

If these quixotic journeymen seem to reflect his own state of mind, says Jarmusch, "It's true. I love to be in that off-kilter position, of not really knowing how to interpret things. My mind opens up, because I'm trying to imagine what the truth of it is. Which is one of the reasons I'm interested by the theories of Dogme 95. In my own work, I really like the idea of stripping things back down to reevaluate what's needed, as in how do you tell a story? What is cinema? How do you work with certain things? Do you need all the tricks? What do you need?"

Although his inspirations may seem scattered, the plot, attests Jarmusch, "Has never been of first importance to me. The characters are. I start with actors whose work I know, or whom I know personally, and create characters from who they are. Then everything else becomes kind of like making a connect-the-dots drawing. I'm a real detail freak. I know every ashtray, every article of clothing, what kind of cigarette they smoke, what kind of car they drive, the shoes they wear. All those things end up creating the atmosphere of the film. I keep on collecting things that may seem disparate but I just keep on collecting if they have some vague connection to the kind of world I'm thinking the story will eventually take place in."

The forty-six-year-old's own training as a savvy film disciple began when his mother—a film reviewer for Ohio's *Akron Beacon Journal*—used to drop him off on Saturdays at the cinema, where the young teenager would drown in double-features. After a brief stint as a journalism major at Northwestern University— "tossed out," he laughs—he later graduated from Columbia University and then wandered off to Paris for a year. Returning to New York, with no prior film experience, he was accepted into the NYU film school where he was hired as Nicholas Ray's teaching assistant. The two became close friends.

It was Nick Ray in fact, says Jarmusch, who passed on what became an important corollary to the young filmmaker, when he compared acting to piano playing. "He said, 'The dialogue is in the left hand, the melody is in the eyes.' He was right. When I came back from Japan, I came back with a load of videotapes that I couldn't find in the States that, of course, had no subtitles. But believe me, if you watch an Ozu film, subtitled or not, you more than understand. Language is very important, but it is not necessarily the primary way of knowing what someone is feeling. Actors are expressing a lot of things through many tiny things, not just the language."

To date, Jarmusch still finds himself most inspired by the personal visions of European filmmakers. Although, he adds sweetly, "I also like big Hollywood entertainments. Sometimes, just sometimes, they are actually good. Sure, there are those American filmmakers who have a strong personal vision that comes across in their work, but the American system is not really nurturing that. And certainly in other cultures, like in China and India, there is a different sense of using the narrative form as a form of expression, as an art form versus purely a product for the market. For my part, when I used to get an idea that was directly connected to something in another film or book, I'd keep it away, and say that's not original. But I am changing, somewhat." Or perhaps he is beginning a new tradition? "Perhaps...Seijan Suzuki, who, although he is quite old now, hopes to be preparing a new film. When I showed *Ghost Dog* to him he said, 'Ah, you steal from me, I will steal from you.' And I said, 'I would be proud. I would be honored.'"

> **"The argument** between digital video and film is no argument. Film is better. It's better, it's better, it's better."
> **JAMES GRAY** / Writer/director, *Little Odessa, The Yards*

**Off the top of your head, what do you find most frightening?**

> Earthquakes. They really scare me. I was in one in L.A. and one in Tokyo. In the Tokyo one, it was really crazy. I woke up in a hotel room with this lamp hanging from the ceiling swinging back and forth. You couldn't open a window, which is pretty unpleasant, so you are sealed in this kind of swaying coffin.

**Your work reflects a strong affinity for music.**

> I love music. I pretty much listen to music all the time, but especially when I'm starting to write and getting ideas. I think it inspires me more than literature and movies and everything put together in a way. I was a musician in the late '70s early '80s. What band, you ask? Well, I would rather not divulge that information. Let's just say we played a lot in New York and opened for a lot of English bands like Echo and the Bunnyman and the Psychedelic Furs. Me and another guy wrote most of the vocals. Mostly I played oddly tuned guitars, a tiny Casio, did some pre-sampling stuff and some very primitive keyboards that used some early Moog synthesizers.

**Do you approach filmmaking in that fashion?**

> There are sculptural, musical elements that I guess I internalize. When you go out to shoot a film with all these people it's physically very demanding. It's almost like you're going through a marble quarry and you're carving a big chunk off the side of the hill, hoisting it down and taking it back. Then when you are in the editing room, you start sculpting it and you might have thought it was a horse, but it turns out to be a moose.
>
> The editing really becomes a way of letting the materials speak to you, telling you "this is what I want to be." When you impose your preconceived ideas rigorously on the material, then it tends to object.

**Especially as an independent filmmaker, do you feel somewhat like a cultural archeologist?**

> Labels don't interest me. I don't know what indie really means anymore anyway. And I'm not a sociologist. My point of view is from a pretty marginal perspective, and my group of friends are pretty much outside the mainstream, to say the least. I do think we are losing the ability to look back and forwards, to look in both directions at the same time, but it's all very subjective. The more advanced the culture gets, the more we look back. The

more I learn about aboriginal cultures and philosophies, for instance, the more respect I have—and the more advanced they seem, although they are labeled primitive.

## Do you wish you could be speedier when you work?

I just do it the way I do it. I don't know any other way. I'm not very ambitious, and I certainly don't want to make a film every year. I do a film when it comes to me. As soon as I'm done with one, I start working on another, but it's not like I'm driven to make a film by the end of every year. Woody Allen, Spike Lee, I don't know how they do it.

I don't really think they own their own production companies, oversee the financing, all the pre-production casting, the writing of the script, directing and then end up in the editing room every day for months and months and months. Woody Allen doesn't even promote his films. That's a half year off your work clock right there.

Anyway, that's the way I do it in order to keep control over the film. I'm very lucky to make films the way I want to, and it means a lot to me to keep making films the way I want. I want to do it for as long as possible, or until they make me stop. Control is very important to me.

## Despite your fascination with Dogme 95, is that why you'd never do a Dogme film? Because you'd have to give up control?

No. For one, just the fact that it is Dogme 95 makes it already passe. I do like it...I like having to stop and think about it. I like the fact that you can break nine of the ten rules, confess to them and still say your film was Dogme, that you were aware of what rules you broke...it has this great tongue-in-cheek element. Even so, I think Dogme, although it is a really interesting idea, it attracts me more as a theory than as a result.

## Have you ever suffered a creative block?

Actually I have. I have a notebook that contains nine notes for nine things, sort of my security notebook, so that I don't think, "Oh man I don't have any ideas—I'm blocked! That's it, I'm finished!" They're not full-fledged stories, they're just collections of ideas of a story, but the last three films I have made have not been made out of those nine stories, so it's like a security book. Who knows? I may never do any of them.

# RICHARD LINKLATER

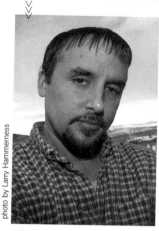

Following his last two features, *SubUrbia*, and the studio-made *The Newton Boys*, Richard Linklater, the Texas-born child of the '60s, has made two fairly low budget, wildly diverse and unconventional films, marking his first forays into digital video.

There is the three-character drama *Tape*, a sly, sharply written, blacker-than-black comedy with real-world sting about truth, justice and sexual consent, starring Ethan Hawke, Uma Thurman and Robert Sean Leonard. At the other end of the playing field is *Waking Life*, a philosophical, animated adventure that harks back to the filmmaker's elliptical *Slacker*.

*Waking Life's* dreamy *mise en scene* follows a *Candide*-like character (Wiley Wiggins of Linklater's *Dazed and Confused*) who, in a "waking dream," enters into dialogues with everyday humanity in pursuit of the meaning of life. A collaboration with Bob Sabiston and Tommy Pallotta, the pair responsible for several animated shorts, including *Roadhead*, the film was shot on DV with a one-chip camera and animated by Sabiston and a team of animators with "interpolated rotoscoping," a technique which allows artists to digitally redraw live-action footage.

Was pushing the creative envelope with technological invention enough to send him screaming back to the high budget pleasures of 35mm and his Airstream trailer? As Linklater tells it, who knows what dreams may come...

## What was the concept behind *Waking Life*?

Well, with *Dazed and Confused* I was really trying to capture the teenage mindset of being fourteen years old and all the complexity of trying to understand the world. I remember me and my friends, we didn't feel like we were stupid, we had that pseudo-philosophical thing going, and I guess I've always thought a lot about identity and self and a lot of those fundamental questions. I remember as a kid asking a teenager these questions, and still asking them as an adult, but you never fully get answers for them. The questions are never answered and it's the eternal mystery that you just kind of deal with. You evolve and wrap around those questions, but I also like the idea of the spirit in a world of ideas, all that it conjures. *Waking Life* was a chance for me to delve back into those really rudimentary ideas, to ask, "What am I? And what is the fabric of life?" but from an older perspective.

It is an exploration of something personal in that it incorporated a lot of other people and ideas, but what this movie is about—and I think that what life is about—is that we always think these things, these questions of the world, the odd phenomena that happens to us and are so unique to ourselves, and I knew there would be precedent out there.

**You've said that *Waking Life* is also autobiographical in a way.**

Nothing in the movie takes place in the waking state. It's all a dreamscape. I used the line in the movie, "You're either sleepwalking through your waking world, or 'wake-walking' through your dreams." It works on a couple of levels: a conscious dream state where you can't be awake in your dreams, that's a possibility, and then there's also your waking life. It's an effort to be more aware in your waking state, awake in your waking state. I like the idea of life being awakened. What I meant by that was that you're in your dreams and you think you're awake so you don't realize that you are in a state potentially where you can experience a much broader range of possibilities. That was the source of a lot of the dialogue and situations in the movie.

Many of the things within the film actually happened to me in lucid dreams. I think there are endless possibilities in lucid dreams. It's a learned process and yet it's something you can't learn. So the story is based on a series of lucid dreams I had over twenty years ago. I had this series of flash awakenings. It went on for a few days, or it seemed liked few days. I tried to capture the spirit of those series of encounters that seemed to go on forever. It got kind of ominous after a while, and I felt trapped; when I did wake up, I'd think, "What is that? I should make a movie about that. This whole film for me was a chance to fully explore that. I did extensive clinical research. Lucid dreaming is a very well documented, academic phenomena. It's a product of sleep. I like it because it seemed very tangible to me. It's not necessarily mystical or religious, it is what you bring to it.

**What is it about the conundrums of spirituality that fascinate you?**

There is always that part of your brain that's examining the world, the nature of everything. I guess I think a lot about identity. That's why the eyes are so important in *Walking Life*. The eyes are the window to the animated soul.

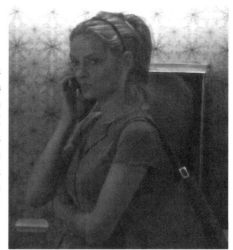

**You mentioned you discovered something rather unusual in your dream research?**

I sure did. There's an institute at Stanford that is the hotbed of this sleep research and they have all these devices that will wake you up when you're asleep; it realizes you're in REM sleep and puts these light flashes on your eyelids. That's how I found out that women who are consciously lucid have an incredibly high rate of orgasms in their dreams, almost 99 percent, a lot more than men. To the female psyche it's a very sensual world. Honestly. It's a fact I came across.

**No wonder fewer women need Viagra....**
**Is that why there is so much floating imagery in the film?**

Maybe. [Laughs] But there is a literal floating/flow aspect throughout the whole movie. I was up in a hot air balloon with helicopters, and there is the floating of the animation itself. For instance, if you have a completely stationary head, talking, it has this breathing, floating, shifting aspect that I thought was really interesting and I thought, that's the way you see things in your imagination. It flows, there really aren't stills in your brain. Which is why I thought rotoscoping was the best way to go.

**The rotoscoping involved thirty-one animation artists who "drew over" the live action footage?**

Bob Sabiston's software is actually a variant of rotoscoping. It allows you to take footage into the software and then over it. That's the easiest way to think of it. The software allows a new way

I think it's a mistake to SHOOT a DV movie like it was a 35mm feature.

to paint that's a combination of tracing and painting. The original imagery is very organic. And the animators are not all computer people or animators but artists, so it was very labor intensive and detailed. It's as creative as what the artist wants to bring to it, and it can be realistic or far out. And in using the rotoscoping you get that extra layer of tension of seeing the real people and words and animating them. I thought it would be really touching to have animated characters who really care a lot about humanity, freedom and about being individuals, while still living in that world of ideas. When you see animated figures, cartoon figures, they're usually geared much more towards comedy and a younger audience. So I thought it would be cool to appeal to both.

**That sounds both dreamy and extremely pragmatic.**

Well, we live in such a material world. If the world wasn't made in seven days, it's all out the window, isn't it? [Laughs]

One hundred and forty years ago Darwin showed us where we came from and we didn't want to hear it because it really lowered the value of our lives. The next generation started to take it as the truth, and some people still deny it today because it makes them feel like we are less. Same thing with dream states. If your deepest feelings and mind-altering experiences can be explained as some manifestation of your brain, it doesn't mean it's not real, and it shouldn't lessen them. As consciousness evolves you can incorporate a lot of science and not take away the true unifying mystical elements that join us all.

**How did you decide to do *Tape*?**

*Tape* was an unproduced play by Stephen Belber that Ethan Hawke sent to me. I don't read a lot of things, and it's rare I see something that really gets into me. I guess it was the ambiguity, the thoughts of memory and the way it concerns an incident that happened ten years ago and how it still affected their lives. The possibilities seemed endless. It is a one-act play, only sixty pages, so there was some concern that it wouldn't be long enough, but would instead be a little featurette. But it was the tightest thing I'd ever read. I think the problem of an adaptation of a play is over-theatricality; you get that stage-bound feeling. The challenge was to make it very cinematic, very real, and I think the DV approach really worked well in that way. I think it's a mistake to shoot a DV movie like it was a 35mm feature.

**Were you looking for a project that you and Ethan could do together?**

The thing about working with people like Ethan again is that you know them, you think a lot alike. So we're good collaborators. Ethan brings a lot of energy to it. He did a little scene in *Waking Life,* and that was the first thing we worked on since *Before Sunrise,* which was a special creative experience. We're two guys who like to sit around all day and talk about what we're doing, talk about character, and dig in and work that way. It's a very cerebral process and I think we enjoy each other's process.

**Did you shoot *Tape* yourself?**

Yep. Just me and Maryse Alberti. It was fun. At a certain point all the stuff that comes with doing a multimillion dollar film, the trailer and studio and everything that comes with it; it all gets in the way. As a filmmaker I always think about how I'd like to rehearse it and get it perfect and then shoot it. This is the closest we can come to this process. Usually actors are fitting into the apparatus of the filmmaking, whereas this is an apparatus that wraps around the performances and I think that's very freeing for the actors. They were confined in the way the characters are there, but there's a lot going on in that room. I like that tension. It was amazing to dance around the room, to cover these people, to know them from the soles of their feet to the palms of their hands.

**You were working on *Tape* while *Waking Life* was being edited. What was that like?**

Double your pleasure, double your fun—that's what it was like. They're so damn different! It's like showing two sides of my brain. *Tape* came about rather quickly in the animation process of *Waking Life. Waking Life* was the big one. *Tape* was shot in a week, rehearsed for two, and happened pretty quickly, although the post-production took forever, like any film. But they both came to finish line at the same time. I did the sound mixes actually one week after each other.

**Why did you choose for these two films to be your first foray into digital filmmaking?**

In DV, because you can do it within a lower budget, you really can do something more personal, more experimental. Also, I had been thinking about doing something digitally for a while. Although we shot *Waking Life* digitally, we could've shot it in anything. It didn't really matter, because it was all done in the computer. But once we fed it into the computer and all the images were digitized, it loosened me up stylistically and made me think how neat or cool it would be to shoot a whole movie with these cameras and that led me to *Tape*. I thought, yeah, we can just shoot that digitally and that would be a way to make this into a movie.

I think shooting those two movies was fun. That's the big thing. It's fun to operate the camera yourself. Using DV, you could keep it rolling and document everything. Burn that tape, baby, burn! Document everything! Use that camera! Working digitally offers a greater immediacy, and it really has loosened me up stylistically. With bigger movies, there's just so much involved, and it's not quite as intimate. It became all about the acting. What about that for a trend?

"**I think Dogme** is great. It forces you to be more creative with other aspects of moviemaking. The digital thing only increases that. I've been a making a digital movie with a friend of mine for five years and I've always agreed it heightens the reality. It's almost as if you're watching the news. It stimulates the sense of something being documented. ❖ It's a lot more freeing when you're being filmed as well. It's not this like huge formal set-up. I was actually going to make a digital film with a friend of mine, Adam Goldberg, who made this film called *Scotch and Milk*. The concept was to use video to blur the line between reality and fiction as much as possible. Not in the Dogme sense. My wife is going to play my girlfriend and we're going to set up all these fictional scenarios in our own lives, trying to find the ultimate self-expression. I guess through a certain process the ultimate self-expression is turning the camera on and leaving it on all day. Put a tape over the red light and just live, forgetting it. Living there within a story or within a scenario or a theatrical concept. Not necessarily to expose our lives onto a movie, but to get the nuances of what it is to discuss something within our personal lives and have that revealed. ❖ Whether it is true to our relationship or isn't, it is more possible if you just forget the camera's on and start living. You start becoming less conscious of the fact that millions of people are going to be watching you. I think it comes from a less homogenized place. ❖ It's true, though. Life is becoming much more like docu-life. My father used to not let us watch television and when I started acting I realized that I'd started behaving like they do in sitcoms, or like some executive production producer's concept of the way I should be living, because I was watching these TV shows. That was freaky."

**GIOVANNI RIBISI** / Actor, *Saving Private Ryan, The Gift*

# GUS VAN SANT

>>>

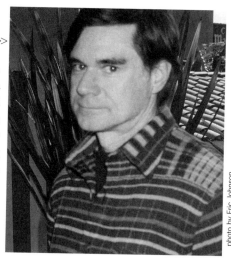

Originally a painter, Gus Van Sant, forty-eight, began making shorts in the early '70s at the Rhode Island School of Design, where schoolmates included David Byrne and other members of Talking Heads. Falling under the influence of avant-garde directors such as Stan Brakhage, the Kuchar brothers, Jordan Belson, Jonas Mekas and Andy Warhol, the Louisville, Kentucky, native made *Alice in Hollywood* (1981), about a naïve young actress who abandons her ideals, but couldn't get it released. Scraping together $25,000 with money saved from his job at a New York advertising agency, he debuted with the black-and-white feature, *Mala Noche* (1985), a tale of luckless love between a gay liquor store clerk and a Mexican immigrant, and hasn't stopped making movies since.

Whether following four Portland, Oregon, addicts who rob pharmacies to feed their habits in *Drugstore Cowboy* (1989), charting the career arc of a murderously ambitious weathergirl in *To Die For* (1995), riding the mainstream with the hugely popular Oscar®-winner *Good Will Hunting* (1997), executing his shot-for-shot remake of the Alfred Hitchcock's classic *Psycho*, or going back to college for his most recent project, *Finding Forrester*, Van Sant always finds a way to keep his absurdist universe roiling with demented romantics and disenfranchised idealists.

**The man who made *Mala Noche* directing Sean Connery: that's pretty anarchic.**

That's true; Sean is not exactly your independent film actor. I was around eleven when I saw my first James Bond movie. I knew I was directing an icon, but he was very easy. I usually try to get the actor to do what he is most comfortable doing. For whatever reason, we saw eye to eye on everything. I agreed with what he said, and vice versa.

**Will your fans find *Finding Forrester* too commercial?**

My people...? [In a robot voice] My people will think what I want them to think. Actually, I don't think I have people, hidden away somewhere. I'm really not positive of that. If you list all my films, the truth is, they are heading in that commercial vein, but also sort of stubbornly staying outside what one would think is the general, accessible Hollywood movie. But the reason I'm saying all of this is that what you get in your head is that it's easy to make a mainstream film—you just follow the formula. The first time I sort of did something like this was in *Good Will Hunting*. I've never actually talked to other filmmakers about this, but I'd always wanted to test the theory and with *Good Will Hunting*, I actually got to, and it turned out really well.

**So you never worried about selling out?**

When I was poor I was trying desperately to sell out to anybody. Before *Drugstore Cowboy*, I was working as a temporary secretary. I was doing advertising commercials, public service announcements, things like that in Portland on a $500 budget, making $100 for myself. In a good week I'd make $25. I was selling my books to make the rent.

**And now?**

Filmmakers that are coming from a noncommercial arena generally stick with it. After you do your first film you don't generally go commercial. If you list *Mala Noche, Drugstore Cowboy, Private Idaho, Even Cowgirls Get the Blues* and *To Die For*—the latter being the most commercial—yes, they were heading in that direction.

Even so, *To Die For* which was made at Columbia Studios, had very low status among the executives, which was a good thing because even in a studio way it was an outside, artistic thing as opposed to commercial work.

When I looked at *Good Will Hunting*, it was obviously a straight ahead, commercial type of story, the kind I liked in the 1970s when I was learning about film. I used to really like those kinds of movies. They were made in a different kind of Hollywood and it has metamorphosed to a place where they no longer make those types of movies because they aren't as accessible to as many people as an action movie is.

**You've been interested in shooting in video for a while, haven't you?**

During *Cowgirls* I had a little Sony, a nondigital camera, and I shot [producer] Lori Parker's baby in a crib to see what it was like to blow it up to 35mm, to see if it was possible. We could've done it.

**Your first foray into digital filmmaking is _Easter_,
one part of an omnibus project written by
Harmony Korine. How did that come about?**

The project is called _Jokes_ and mine is about an albino couple
who live in a black community and the man of the house decides
that he's gay. They still have to make the other two sections that
Harmony wrote. He's been waiting forever. But it all began when
I saw the Dogme 95 film _The Celebration_. I was really excited and
inspired by that kind of ability, and the idea back-to-basics filmmaking. Then I saw a rough cut of _julien donkey-boy_, and thought
the idea was really taken to another level by Harmony and
Anthony Dod Mantle.

I wanted to do all these little cameras, like in _julien_, but
Anthony didn't want to do that. He really wanted to shoot on
film. Somehow I talked him into shooting digital on Sony
PD100. I got a taste of that and then I went back into traditional 35mm on a dolly for _Finding Forrester_.

**Why were you drawn to DV?**

Because it's super cheap. Film just seems to cost at least
$30,000, but for $3000—less if you get used equipment—you
can shoot unlimited amounts of footage in synch and make
whatever you want. The quality is much better than it was five
years ago.

**What do you think about the new 24P HD
cameras?**

I haven't played with HD, but it seems like having a Polaroid on
the set—whatever is on the screen is what you're going to get.
Technical guesswork is going to be gone. I think that's definitely the next wave. Those HD cameras even have the potential to
emulate the cinema flicker.

**Did you find yourself working in the "stripped
down" Dogme style?**

Clearly, _Easter_ wasn't a Dogme film, but in doing something
smaller I actually got to do a little of what I've been trying to do
since _Drugstore Cowboy_. On _Mala Noche_, we had a crew of three—DP,
sound person and our PA and me. I missed that. I saw this documentary where Ingmar Bergman was shooting and they had
only five or six people on the set. I don't see why it's not possible to work like that more often. Money probably has something
to do with it. We did have a crew of only fifteen people, which is

something I'd been trying to do since *Drugstore Cowboy,* and failed at it then. For *My Own Private Idaho,* I insisted on having a twenty-person crew, which meant ten people on the set, and ten people in the office. It seemed like an impossibility with the way we were being funded, which I thought was absurd. We ended up with a thirty-person crew, which is still pretty small.

I think that in using small crews the key is to multitask people, and not divide them into departments. They're like those Navy SEALs who can do ten different things. They're demolition experts and they can do sound! That's the way they tend to work in Europe, where crews have always been smaller.

**Did that hands-on approach work for you on *Easter*?**

Yes and no. When I shot, I started not to pay attention to the camera I was using as much as I was to the action, so I got out of focus and Anthony got very, uh, brisk. My editor on *Finding Forrester,* Valdis [Oskarsdottir, also the editor on *julien* and *The Celebration*] who also worked on *Easter,* doesn't like it when something is out of focus either. People working in Copenhagen get really annoyed when things are out of focus.

But what worked for me, shooting digitally, was the less-is-more part, getting rid of all the departments. It's more organic, less corporate, less of a Hollywood process.

**What else did you learn working in DV?**

I found out that I don't know that much about it, but also I found out they don't know that much either. That's what I learned from Anthony. I assumed he would just blast in and be like, "Okay, this is how you do it." That was kind of naive of me, because the technology changes minute by minute. There isn't just one way to do it.

Anthony had a model of camera like the camera they used to shoot *The Celebration.* I asked what happened to the actual *Celebration* camera. It was just a rental and went back into the pool of cameras. I asked, "why isn't it in a museum or something? Why don't you have it?"

Anyway he didn't want to shoot that way again, he wanted to do something new. So we were shooting with three chip cameras that were bigger and he didn't particularly know them. He knew lots of things about them, and a lot from the other cameras, and he was sort of fiddling around because he always had to learn anew because the bigger cameras can do different things than the little cameras.

I mean this is a film cinematographer who's playing with a weird medium, the prosumer tools where the guy at home knows as much as the DP, because they're not made for technicians. You really just kind of play around. Anthony could get really lost in the camera and work it for hours, shooting a tree or something like that because there were all these things it could do. I wanted to buy one from the rental house but Anthony said, "You don't want that camera. We'll blow a lot of hours with it, and after 200 hours the camera is basically unusable anyway. The heads wear out, and it's too expensive to put new heads on the camera because it only costs $1,500 to begin with. You don't replace the heads—you just buy a new camera." I didn't know that.

**Musicians say that you don't get the full tone one can get if one goes the digital route. Is it the same with digital video?**

We recorded our sound on tape for *Finding Forrester*, also on *Easter* and *Good Will Hunting*. Pretty much all the films we're sticking with analog tape, although we didn't do that for *Psycho*. The mixer really liked the warm tone that you can get if you manipulate a voice recording on digital. You might as well record it on analog; it's just smoother, sort of mellow, not as hyper. I think that's probably true of film as well. Film images are hazier and more powdery and more mellow as well. I think if you get to a certain stage, the digital can mimic the quality or run it through a film path where you go to film and back to digitally manipulating things to get a different quality.

**So, it's only digital video for you from now on?**

Not really. I want to figure out other ways to go about it. You could make up your film as you go like Mike Leigh, or even the way Spike Lee does it. I want to make sure whatever it is I'm doing, that I'm really attracted to that concept.

When Lars von Trier and Thomas Vinterberg started with DV, those guys had made previous films that are really good. I remember Thomas' *The Boy Who Walked Backwards* and Lars' *Zentropa*; both are really polished, traditional cinematic storytelling. When those guys started to fool around with DV, they were actual filmmakers who started playing with that medium as opposed to people who knew nothing about it.

I'm currently under the influence of these Hungarian film-makers Bela Tar and Laszlo Krasznahorkai. They did this film called *Satan's Tango*. Oh my God. It was a combination of Sam Beckett, Andrei Tarkovsky and Andy Warhol. They shoot in black-and-white and let the camera just run, with practically ten minute takes. It is really the other side of the universe to the digital revolution and I'm really interested in that, too. I don't know what I want to spend my time doing next. I like the idea of spending time doing it and figuring it out—so it could be DV or it could be film.

**Do you think only people who understand filmmaking should try DV?**

No. That's a personal decision. A person who's actually shooting is learning right then. It's hard to learn when you're only planning. You can write screenplays and plan things out, but when you really learn is when you start running the camera, and whatever is supposed to be happening is happening. Then you play it back and evaluate what you shot. It's the process of shooting and playing back and showing other people, grabbing somebody from down the street and showing them the thing. With this trial and error process, you actually learn. If kids have that ability to grab a camera and start working, then they start learning and inventing their own processes.

**You seem to always be learning. Chris Doyle, your DP on *Psycho*, said that the film was your way of getting Hollywood to fund an anarchic art project.**

I had the idea to remake *Psycho* from the very first time I got into a meeting at Universal with *Drugstore Cowboy*. The only reason they actually accepted the concept is because I made money on *Good Will Hunting* and they thought it might end up being like a *Scream*. Maybe it seemed like I was selling out at the time, but I was doing completely the opposite. It was kind of an appropriation that I had never really seen done on film before and it seemed to have an application in the commercial medium. But, it was a full-on experiment, a Frankenstein, a genetic experience.

The money I was to make on *Psycho* was more money than if you were to take my entire life and combine it all together, and for the biggest art project of my life! But, it became clear that if you did it literally shot by shot, you destroyed what you were cre-

ating. You'd kill it
by being too rigid,
because ultimately it
has its own life, but
appropriation was
always one of the big
things we did in art

The MONEY I was
to make on *Psycho*
was more money
than if you were
to take my ENTIRE
*Life* and combine
it all together,
and for the
biggest ART project
of my life!

school. Marcel Duchamp was the originator of this kind of thing.
Warhol did the same, for instance with the Campbell's Soup can.
It's all a part of the pop glamour myth.

**With all the input you get, do you ever feel there
is too much information in the world in the sense
that too many collages of other people's images
work their way into your brain?**

I don't really look at lot of images. I don't watch TV; I don't go
on the Web. I look at magazines if I'm travelling, but I wouldn't
say overcome with images. If you're just living normally,
depending on how many movies you might see in a week or how
many newspapers or magazines you're reading, that's pretty
much already. But I don't think I'm unduly influenced by anything. I think I did that when I was younger. I did sort of indulge
in a lot of images and things, but I don't any more.

**You went to film school with Talking Heads
at RISD?**

They were a year ahead of me. I went to their first show. At the
time there were something like ten people in the band and David
Byrne sang *Psycho Killer,* but he didn't have all the words so they did
some Velvet Underground songs too. It's weird how all these
musicians go to art school. I guess there's nowhere else for rock
stars to go, unless they go to traditional music schools, but people like that tend to be more into multimedia, pop art and culture. I had a band [Kill All Blondes] in the '80s, for all of about
half a year. Some of the albums are actually available on
Amazon.com now, which is pretty funny. The band was also an
experiment. I wanted to see if I would crack under pressure
onstage, which I was very afraid of. But I can actually handle it. I
am proud to say I remembered all the lyrics.

**Do you get those kinds of jitters as a filmmaker?**

No. Mostly because you are the one in control, whether you like
it or not. A film set is usually a pretty friendly place. You can be

shy, domineering, whatever, but the key is to know what you want, or else it quickly devolves into mutiny. I like to bring it right to that edge. When I get there I know that everybody expects me to make that decision and I wait...and wait...and wait...and they start feel like I don't know what I actually want. And sometimes, if you wait long enough, somebody will come up with a better idea, and then you get to use that idea. It's like playing poker, you want to hold out as long as possible.

## AGNES VARDA

Behind the hotel room door, a voice urgently announces, "I am coming! A moment...." The door whips open and a petite woman in her early her seventies, crowned with a shiny cap of dark red hair, leans up on tiptoe and kisses me on either cheek.

"Bonjour! I am Agnes Varda, and you are here to see me, yes? Would you like some tea? It is cold out, no? I have a cold," she says without a pause in heavily accented English, marching me into the living room, past the poster for her latest film, the documentary *The Gleaners and I.* "It's a beautiful poster, no? Put the chair next to the couch, I make you your tea." She sneezes spasmodically, sighs, then raises up a large atomizer and sprays herself liberally from all directions. A halo of scented mist forms around her head. "It is only roses," she whispers, enraptured, her eyes closed. "I love the smell. For a moment it takes me away, to my garden at home."

Varda's documentary was partially inspired by Jean-Francois Millet's 1857 painting "The Gleaners" depicting three women gathering sheaves and kernels in a wheat field. The painting propelled Varda into the countryside to study the history of the gleaners—those who clean up what's left after the harvest—as well their urban variants, the citybound scavengers who subsist on the leftovers and castoffs of modern society. Shot on digital video, *The Gleaners and I* is a humorous, personal memoir as well as a discourse on poverty and the traditional right to scavenge in French history and culture; ideas that are movingly underscored by scenes of a magistrate in full regalia standing in a cabbage field and citing the royal edict establishing the right to glean, a hilarious seaside argument about oysters, and a dog adorned with a boxing glove.

Unusual counterpoints perhaps, but Varda has always followed her own cinematic path. Moving effortlessly between documentary and narrative filmmaking, with a preference for subjects that emphasize, "the confusion of the world of objects, caught between the material world and culture," her work has an extraordinary stylistic freedom and is an unapologetic exploration of auteurist will. Married for nearly thirty years to the late filmmaker Jacques Demy (*The Umbrellas of Cherbourg, The Young Girls of Rochefort, Donkey Skin*), and affectionately referred to as the "grandmother of the New Wave," Varda cut her teeth as the official photographer for Jean Vilar's productions at the Theatre National Populaire. Impatient to make her first feature, but lacking a government subsidy or approval, she made *La Pointe Courte* (1954), a low-budget effort (edited by landmark New Waver Alain Resnais) about a young couple's marital problems in a Mediterranean fishing village. She made several short films before her next features, *Cleo From 5-7* (1961) and *Le Bonheur* (1965); two decades later, showed she had lost none of her fire with the much admired *Vagabond* (1985), a riveting look at events leading to the death of a young drifter played by Sandrine Bonnaire.

Her 1976 film *One Sings, The Other Doesn't,* made at the height of the women's movement, prompted one (male) critic to proclaim it "The only truly woman's film so far made."

"It is a paradox, how I work. I am a very passionate person, but I am also a strict editor. To achieve what I need as an artist, I like to work on my own images, fantasies and associations, and to be free minded," she says, lounging on the couch, curling her freshly pedicured feet beneath her. "But," she adds, referring to the subjects of her latest effort, "because I knew these people were fragile and not easy to approach, I had to wait, to make them come to me." She smiles serenely. "I was patient like an angel." She sits up suddenly and sprays herself and most of the room with more rosewater. "I am so jet-lagged. It's getting late, no? I will get dressed. I am in New York! I want to go the museums. I want to see the city! It is cold outside?" Without waiting for a response,

> **"Von Trier has** become such a DV proselytizer that he ignores the medium's expressive limitations. Until DV technology vastly improves, I'll stick with Brian De Palma, who remarked in his press conference for *Mission to Mars* that DV was best used by novice directors who no longer have to wait five years for someone to take a chance on their projects."
>
> **AMY TAUBIN** / Journalist, *Village Voice*

Varda picks up the atomizer and heads into the bedroom to dress. I hear the sound of manic spritzing and a long exhaled sigh.

"Where others see a cluster of junk, I see a cluster of opportunity," salvage artist Louis Pont says in *The Gleaners,* a point of view that continues to be Varda's modus operandi towards life. "I am not making a career, I am making films," she explains. "I don't have to make a statement or take a philosophical approach. These people speak for the facts. They speak to how some people can be so generous to others even more destitute than they. Some people shine!" she exults, "And, having met some of these poor people shining for me, it makes me feel so good."

Without even buttoning her coat Varda hastily exits the hotel with me in tow, pausing momentarily, her eyes darting hither and thither, soaking in the noise, the lights, the buildings, the onrushing crowd. "Ah...wonderful. What pleasure! I wish I had one of my little digital cameras!" she exclaims, and heedlessly jumps the curb, winding through the dangerously trafficked road. Varda looks back over her shoulder, "Come! This way! Follow me!" The Grandmother of the New Wave beckons as she is swallowed by the stream of humanity.

## Why did you choose to work with these digital cameras?

The intimacy, remembering the shooting I did years ago with this little camera I had. I would have to keep rewinding it because it would last only fifty seconds. It was a totally amateur camera and I made a short from that in 1958. I was approaching people in the street, but not speaking with them. It is a theme I have been following all my life.

It always takes a little thinking to decide what is the best technique for the purpose of your film, not just the chic or fashionable thing to do or have. So using the digital camera was equivalent in a way.

We used thirty minutes from my own camera. I have a tripod which is very light, and another camera head with which I could do panoramic shots, smooth images if I needed them. I liked to mix it up. The rest of the time I had a DP who used a bigger DV camera, like you see on the news.

I could approach these people and not look like a filmmaker, be in the mix. In that way they forget you are there. For *The Gleaners and I,* I could not have done it another way. I myself shot, which enriched the film with my sincerity, I hope, or at least it was a way of saying I'm there. I could never have asked a cameraman, "Can you come and film a close-up of my hand?" I would-n't like that. I like very much the feeling of being myself and being a filmmaker who is seeing myself. In this way, one hand is filming while the other is acting. It is interesting—as an artist you are always working with instant feeling, suffering. On the other hand you have to be a rigorous editor and very strict in your mind so that you can make an edit that has a meaning that is linked to other elements.

What I am looking for with this film is to touch people, and to touch them somewhere that they don't expect to be touched. In this film I wanted to achieve something quite different, namely to approach a very serious fact of society in which we find out there are people living on the leftovers we throw away. It is a kind of shameful feeling when you see these people, but I want-ed to make a film where the energy of life and the life of these people, their good sense, along with my sense of being a film-maker came out. That is the pleasure of the film, even though it deals with a very difficult subject. That is the paradox I wanted to achieve.

**Did you have any fears in approaching this project?**

Not really, but if you want to speak about problems, I'm afraid to lose my vision. My eyes are fine, now, but...and my memory, now *that* is a disaster!

**Did you miss working with celluloid?**

I love to touch celluloid. I love the smell. The time when you are splicing is good for the mind.

Somebody once asked what do you do with the leftovers of the editing. When we used film, there would be a pile of stock, so people could come and look, but now it's so abstract, because we edit on the Avid. There is nothing in the machine. It is just a program. On the Avid, we did make a program of what we kept and we have the cassette of the shooting, but it doesn't give the feeling that there are any real leftovers. You can't touch it.

It wasn't so hard to adapt to this method, though. I trans-ferred at GTC, in France, where I have been working for more than forty years.

**Will you continue to work digitally?**

It's a new toy, it's like a friend. But as a toy it's very nice to play with, but it's only a tool. Everyone thinks because it is so quick and light, everything is then easier. I don't agree with that. A lot of film festivals, they ask will I do this short piece or the other. I could do the light, do a leaf, I could film my feet and have fifteen students watching me, to learn from everything I do? So, I told them, the camera is just a camera. What is important is what you want to film. You could be like Andy Warhol, and do what he used to do. He left the camera turned on all the time like a tape recorder. That is okay if that's what you want to do, but I didn't feel inspired.

**What do you feel is provocative filmmaking?**

Now, in France there are fifteen new films every Wednesday. It's easy to forget the rest. I did like von Trier's *The Idiots* very much. When Kubrick's *2001* was released, I didn't like that too much at the time, or his *Clockwork Orange.* I hated that film. I remember that Catherine Deneuve and I went together, both of us pregnant without men, watching *Clockwork Orange*—after twenty minutes, we were gone. I didn't want the baby growing inside me seeing such horror.

I like the avant-garde of the '50s. I like that period very much.

**In regard to that, what is your opinion of the current *Cahiers du Cinema*?**

I like them but most of the time I don't understand what they write. But honestly, my feeling is, when you like something, you add something to it when you discuss why you like it. When you spend a lot of time criticizing something, you are wasting time. That is why I find critical discussions of cinema on the whole to be very boring.

## WIM WENDERS

Son of a surgeon, Wim Wenders was born on the 14th of August, 1945, in Düsseldorf, Germany. After high school, he began his studies in medicine (1963-64) and philosophy (1964-65) in Munich, Freiburg and Düsseldorf. He interrupted his education and moved to Paris in October 1966, where he studied painting and worked as an engraver in an atelier in Montmarte. He returned to Germany in 1967, worked briefly in the Düsseldorf office of United Artists and entered the Graduate School of Film and Television, which had just been founded in Munich.

Wim Wenders graduated from the Hochschule with his first feature film *Summer in the City*, but he really began his professional career in 1971 with his next film, *The Goalie's Fear of the Penalty Kick*, based on Peter Handke's book of the same name. In 1971, in collaboration with twelve other film-makers, he began a production and distribution company called Film-verlag der Autoren. In 1976, he started Road Movies Filmproduktion in Berlin, which, since 1984, has been run exclusively by Wenders and his producer, Chris Sievernich. Producing and directing through these various companies, Wenders—combining his love of documentary and narrative features—became one of the major figures of the New German Cinema.

In 1977 he directed Dennis Hopper in *The American Friend* (adapted from Patricia Highsmith's novel), which brought him to the attention of Francis Ford Coppola. At Coppola's invitation, he came to the United States in 1978 to shoot *Hammett*, which, along with other work, occupied him until 1982. During this period Wenders made *Lightning over Water* (together with his friend, director Nicholas Ray), followed by *The State of Things*, which won the Golden Lion at the Venice Festival of 1982.

In 1987, besides the release of his film *Wings of Desire* (winner of Best Director prize at 1987's Cannes Film Festival) he also published his first book, *Written in the West*, reflecting his fascination with the American West. This collection of photographs would be followed by other books—collections of essays, reflections on filmmaking, other photo and art books, companion books to his films and more. From 1991 to 1996 he was the appointed Chairman of the European Film Academy and was subsequently elected as its president, but it never held him back from his work behind the camera.

Since the early 1990s, Wenders has filmed his movies mainly in the U.S. and in English, filling the decade with projects such as *Until the End of the World*, a documentary film on fashion designer Yohji Yamamoto; *Beyond the Clouds*, a collaboration with Michelangelo Antonioni; as well as *Far Away, So Close; Lisbon Story, A Trick of the Light* and *The End of Violence*. He kicked off the 21st Century with *The Million Dollar Hotel* and a new project, an American family saga written by *Paris, Texas* collaborator Sam Shepard, tentatively titled *In America*, which he calls, "a true road movie."

Despite his on and off love affair with the critics, Wenders' 1998 award-winning DV documentary *Buena Vista Social Club* gave audiences much to celebrate. Coming from a world player such as Wenders, the richly-lensed, tightly-edited *Buena Vista's* commercial and artistic success gave a leg up to DV's global credibility. For Wenders, it is a filmmaking revolution, a democratizing tool that he believes will turn the industry upside down.

**Do you think the interest in the DV aesthetic is emerging for a particular cultural/political reason?**

Yes! The miniDV cameras are really great weapons for movie-guerillas of all sorts of colors.

**The completed *Buena Vista Social Club*—an all-digital production—went to a transfer company to be burned onto film. So what's the point of all this new technology?**

Good question. It's a giant investment for movie theaters to be equipped with data projectors capable of showing high-resolution product, but that's just a question of time. Right now, too many people still earn a lot of money with the celluloid technology, not just Kodak and Fuji, but all the labs in the world. Only when the advertising industry understands the advantage of digital projection in theaters and how it will improve their business—they can show different ads in the afternoon and at night, different ads at the matinees and at late night shows, one ad before the G-rated movie another before the PG or R-rated ones. If the sun is shining outside, they show the car commercial for the convertible, when it's raining they show the one featuring the sedan, etc. You will see the arrival of data projectors over the next five years.

**What do you think of Lars von Trier's back-to-basics Dogme initiative? Would you find value in utilizing Dogme 95 for a project of yours?**

I loved and admired the Dogme initiative. I can easily imagine shooting by their rules. I discussed it with Lars and told him that my only problem is that I could not add music afterwards. He laughed and said I should just break that rule. Dogme did a lot of good to contemporary filmmaking, and even if it wasn't all that new an approach—Italian neo-realism followed the same credo—it opened a whole new, younger audience to a different kind of filmmaking, smack dab in the middle of the '90s, when "entertainment" ruled. I think Dogme was first and foremost a great marketing tool. I say that without any cynicism, only admiration. It gave low-budget filmmaking an ethos that it had lost.

Pessimists worry that digitalization spells the end of celluloid. I am neither with the pessimists, nor part of the Utopians. I am just an optimist. In the '80s and '90s we saw the decline of everything that was "small, but beautiful." Especially in the movie industry, everything that was small was dwarfed even more. Auteur films, documentaries, critical essays, B-movies as such, films shot in "foreign languages," films for minorities, etc. With the rise of digital technology, I see a chance for all these (almost) lost forms to come to life again, and even to expand. The tools filmmakers have at hand now are unbelievable, and, for the first time, are compatible with the bigger, "professional" means. I am absolutely certain that we will witness a revolution in this coming decade that will turn the film industry upside down. Potentially, at least, there is a great chance for that democratization, and it's not a utopia. It's already happening.

**Which is harder to direct—sex or violence?**

They are both very easy to direct. As you can quickly verify, the worst directors in the world can do it. As far as sex goes, it is mostly filmed in the absence of a director. Most porn movies seem to just be shot somehow, without directing efforts getting in the way. As for violence, you already need more direction, but again, it's easy. I've done a handful of scenes involving fighting, shooting or killing, and I always felt it was a piece of cake. It was, in fact, *too* easy. Violence in movies is mostly cheap, false, prejudiced and downright ridiculous. Real violence is uglier than in movies, less spectacular, much more arbitrary and without heroes—just victims, on both sides.

On the other hand, if you *really* want to enter the heart of violence, or really explore sex (as opposed to exploiting it), both become difficult and you have to make the greatest effort as a director. Chances are that you will fail. Both subjects have been mishandled so often and so badly that it is almost impossible to tackle them from scratch, with a fresh eye, without falling into any trap or any cliché. It happens every now and then, though.

**Do you see cinema today as an art form?**

Cinema is carrying a heavy burden if you see it as art, because it is never just that. Movies are too popular an artform, too close to entertainment and business, too much integrated into a giant industry to play out their "art" potential. Still, some movies dare to take their link to the arts seriously—to the art of storytelling, the art of representation, the art of writing, to the art of acting or to the art of music. Cinema is the crazy melting pot of all these arts, and by definition never pure, never unspoiled.

I don't use the term "art" anymore. I like to think of myself as a craftsman, an organizer of different professions of artists, and as a storyteller, which is also a craft, in my eyes. "Truth," is the one aspect of any film, be it a big studio production, an independent film or a student movie, which can lift it from being an ordinary and industrial product to something close to any "art." There can be moments of truth in a fiction film where you'd never expect it, whereas a nonfiction film, a documentary, might not show you a single second of "truth." It is such a difficult word even to use. In the realm of contemporary movies, I think, it is considered a four-letter word, although it has five of them. In a time of deep cynicism, like today, and in the age of image-avalanches, "truth" is harder to find than the proverbial needle in the haystack. But don't give up: Sometimes you find it in the weirdest places.

**What are the themes that call to you?**

The truth, and nothing but the truth. I still think that movies are made to explore each and every question we have on our mind. I still consider film a fabulous vehicle to approach a subject, not knowing everything about it beforehand, but to find out what I didn't know yet. I love to see (and make) movies which take people through an experience or make them explore unknown territory, whether of the world or of the soul.

**Why do you think filmmaking is viewed as a romantic profession? Is it because it is linked to a certain kind of truth or risk?**

Very few films actually take risks, and very few care about the truth behind their stories. I think your question is romantic, and a little bit nostalgic. Movies are considered glamorous today because they are linked to being rich and famous.

**As a culture, do we display an appetite for reality matched only by our craving for fantasy?**

The appetite for reality seems to be filled by a lot of pseudo-real products. Reality television, *Big Brother*, infotainment. It seems that we have all been brainwashed over the last decade to understand "cinema" more and more as a tool for fantasy. As much as I think that there is nothing wrong with fantasy and entertainment, I regret that the notion of cinema has shrunk so much, and that nothing, at least for a while, seemed to be acceptable in theaters other than "blockbuster products." I am certain that will change again. I am certain "consumers" will eventually prefer a wider variety on their menus again.

**You've shot films in both film and video—what do you think is special about the video image versus the film image? How does it compare with the new 24P HD?**

It's obvious that digital technology will eventually replace film. If you look around film is already quite an obsolete and anachronistic medium. Where else do you still see 19th Century mechanical and photographic equipment? Digital technologies have changed our lives in so many ways, and they will overtake cinema as well. *Eventually*. The 24P HD is a big step in that direction. It will improve again. I see a great chance, not just a loss.

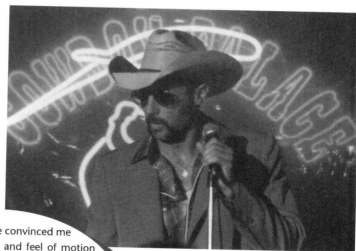

**"The tests** have convinced me that the familiar look and feel of motion picture film are fully present in this digital 24P HD system and that the picture quality between the two is indistinguishable on the large screen."
**GEORGE LUCAS** / Director/Producer/Writer, *THX 1138:4EB, American Graffiti, Star Wars*

>>
>>

*John Gries in Jackpot
(shot in 24P HD).*
courtesy of Mark and Michael Polish
photo by Jo Strettel

## Have filmmakers become too incestuous in their points of view?

I know a lot of filmmakers who live so much in their creations, and have so interiorized the conditions of their jobs and the creative freedom it allows their fantasies, that their actual lives seem to be guided by a complete loss of reality. I see their films more and more feeding on themselves, feeding on other films, no longer influenced by actual experience, only by secondhand experience. That makes a lot of these movies just stillborn in my book.

That's why it is so great to have the chance, every now and then, to stand in the streets with just a camera and a sound man, facing nothing other than blank truth. When you do your next fiction film, you have twenty trucks and a hundred people behind you again. It's good for any filmmaker's mental health to give up this army sometimes and just be out there in the real world. For the audience it is the same. If you only feed on fantasy, if you get addicted to that food and after a while you can't eat anything else, you lose your taste for anything else. And you unlearn that important "difference between seeing and dreaming," to quote you.

## What did you bring from your experience on *Buena Vista Social Club* to *The Million Dollar Hotel*?

There was a certain lightness of being that survived the making of *Buena Vista Social Club* and that carried us through *Million Dollar Hotel*. It was that infectious, contagious energy of those old people and their belief in themselves and their music. *That* was truly an uplifting experience, and I wouldn't want to replace it with any experimental factor or research. In *Buena Vista* we were able to witness something extraordinary, a fairy-tale unfolding in front of our eyes. You can't plan that; you can only be ready for it. Technology always must serve a cause, and not vice versa. Digital technology helped us to catch all the spontaneity of those Cuban musicians—we couldn't have captured the spirit of that film on celluloid.

# DV, AND THE FILM FESTIVALS PRESS

What do top flight critics such as the *New York Times*' Elvis Mitchell, *Variety's* Todd McCarthy, and magazines such as *Premiere, Film Comment* and *Entertainment Weekly,* as well as high profile film festival programmers like Sundance's Geoffrey Gilmore, Toronto's Piers Handling and the New York Film Festival's Richard Peña have in common? They all can in one way or another help make or break a non-star driven feature.

It's an often invisible state of affairs but one which keeps independent filmmakers, distribution executives and even the studios on their toes. Word of mouth, print coverage, showcasing at the right festival—these are all awareness tools, especially for any low budget feature seeking a spot in the limelight. With more and more festivals cropping up, each of them vying for premieres from producers and coverage from the major entertainment sources, the relationships between festivals, the press and distributors is becoming more unsettled and more political than ever before.

Digital video is significant here in that most of the newest low budget features are digital features. The major film festivals, anxious to bring in the riskier independent features, have foregone their previous film-only policy, and are even making it easy for filmmakers by providing digital projection. This means that cash-strapped indies can screen at a major festival such as Sundance before coughing up the rather large fee to transfer to 35mm. Let the ardent distributor help cover that cost! This development has been a major boon to filmmakers who can now produce a feature for significantly less money.

But the debuting filmmakers only get so far. Film-focused publications such as *Res, Filmmaker* and even the *New York Times* have done their share of awareness raising, but the press still needs to do more in terms of validating unusual imagery and helping explain the transition.

The DV versus celluloid battle is still somewhat of a schoolyard skirmish. There is no need to choose one over the other, especially when such wonders can be achieved in both, or in a fusion of the two. A film like Stephen Soderbergh's *Traffic* would be an excellent example of that ethos. But how DV filmmaking techniques will change the aesthetics and language of cinema is an issue both the festivals and the press need to help convey to larger audiences. Aside from the often quoted success of DV auteurs such as Lars von Trier with *Dancer in the Dark*, Mike Figgis' with *TimeCode*, Wim Wenders with *Buena Vista Social Club*, Thomas Vinterberg with *The Celebration*, and even Bennet Miller's indie hit, *The Cruise*, many critics feel celluloid is still far superior, as video will never capture the detail of which film is capable. Furthermore, they are often wary that the widespread ease and use of DV [especially at the hands of neophyte filmmakers] will propel films towards easy captures, unstable setups, inferior image quality and narrative banality. Which is another way of saying that digitization may be good for the flashy bells and whistles of blockbuster movies, but its often uninformed usage spells the end of the art in filmmaking. Much like the computer weakened the craft of writing? Somewhat. Even so, in the right hands, DV can be a wonderful new way to create new stories. And whether it's through the whir of technohappy pixels, or via the sprocketed, chaotic magic of celluoid, both mediums have the ability and the means to tell stories that can move the world. So maybe we all should relax. That is, until a new medium comes along.

# GEOFFREY GILMORE
## Co-Director/Director of Film Programming, Sundance Film Festival

Geoffrey Gilmore has been responsible for film selection and overall programming of the annual festival since 1990. In addition, Gilmore is a programming consultant for the Sundance Film Channel, launched in February of 1996. For fourteen years he served as head of the UCLA Film & Television Archive's programming, and presently he co-teaches a course in the film school on independent production. He is on the board of the Independent Feature Project/West and has served as a consultant for numerous organizations, committees and projects.

### You've been with the Sundance Film Festival for over ten years. What trends have you noticed?

The way to answer that question is by talking about what independent film is now in the process of doing, which is many ways is a process of reinvention, of leaving some of the older genres behind. We used to talk about independent film as having boundaries that were defined by a lack of resources, star power and technology. Now we have films that run the gamut, from films with lots of resources to films done on a shoestring, films that have enormous star power, and films having special effects and animation. The idea of how independent film is evolving is not a question of how it is becoming like a studio film. It's still very script-driven, completely original, still has the ideas and references that make it full and engaging but it is also work that is no longer bound by the old idea of what art cinema was and by the old idea of what the independents were. I think it is more inclusive and more imaginative than it's ever been.

## Is there a digital aesthetic that ghettoizes films shot in this format?

Not on our end. Some distributors want to niche it, but at Sundance we've been working with Betacam in our labs for fifteen years. If someone tells me that high-quality digital projection has existed for the last few years and Sundance has somehow ignored the technology, I'd love to see the evidence. I think what a lot of people have tried to do is suggest that digital represents a specific kind of aesthetic and then showcase it in one particular house. That's the exact opposite of what you should be trying to do. This is a professional format and as a professional format we should be able to showcase it in as many theaters as we have. There is one theater in Salt Lake City, and a theater in Ogden we can't get projectors into, but every single other one we have set up. The digital format should be a transparent thing that blends into the rest of the festival.

Basically I'm saying that every single section, every single program can showcase film in one of three formats—16mm, 35mm or digital. What we're doing this year is offering HD projection in every section of the festival. We've had some digital screenings in the past, and now the digital format is a professional enough format—like 35mm or 16mm—to present movies in. We're not arguing that this is the future, something that may edge out celluloid. We're definitely not announcing that Sundance is now a video festival geared toward television work. All we're saying by offering video projection this year is that the technology has caught up, and it's completely up to the filmmakers to decide how they want to present their work. I'm literally, as this interview is going on, still waiting to hear from four or five films in the festival and whether they'll deliver a 35mm print or go with video projection. Also, remember that it's only recently that we've even had a decent number of digital features to select from. We still didn't get all that many digital submissions this year; nowhere near the numbers people would think, given all the coverage the so-called digital revolution has received. Sundance is about films, not formats.

Many questions surrounding the digital revolution center on this technical presentation, and the digital aesthetic. In the 2001 festival we had twenty-three films that were shot digitally and eighteen that are being projected digitally. In 2000 we projected seventeen films digitally, but a great number of those were films that, for various reasons, might have been finished on film, or were documentaries, or were films that were perhaps shot on Beta and upgraded to HD rather than film. There is prejudice by distributors against releasing DV. Hence, a lot of the films that were shot digitally are not being projected that way. There is still that sense that digital implies not film and that film is still the ultimate quality.

**So it's a matter of content, not format?**

One of the things that is most interesting is that you can't really define what the digital aesthetic is. We are really only beginning to explore it. You can look at DV films that are almost identical to film; you can look at ones that emulate a video look; and there are those that are trying to degrade the image and do something entirely different. For instance, when *The Celebration* first came out, October Films wanted it to be perceived as a "movie" so they initially didn't talk about the DV aspect. All of the attention it received for being shot on a one-chip DV camera came afterwards, when the film was recognized for its content. In *julien donkey-boy* the image is degraded and altered in specific ways—that's an aesthetic choice.

**Do you feel that DV plays with the nature of realism, in regard to its docudrama aspects?**

I wouldn't say it is docudrama. For instance, a film we had in 2001, *Series 7*, is a *Survivor* take off, written long before *Survivor* was ever on the air. It plays with the frame of TV and plays with how that frame sets up our expectations but then it takes you in another direction. In that sense, the ways of understanding what realism and what reality programming are raises different kinds of questions of the imagery you are representing.

## Do you see the influence of the French New
## Wave or Godard on this new crop of filmmakers?

I wish there was! I don't know that I would say there an enormous influence by Godard or, for that matter, a number of different filmmakers. There are certainly a lot of filmmakers here who have seen a lot of different work and may or may not be influenced by that. I don't know if I would say some of the younger ones have branched out as much as they could, and that's something you realize as you meet with people and figure out if they know much about classical Hollywood cinema or European cinema. Yes, in regards to DV, a film can have a kind of a hyper-realism that comes with the form, from the digital aesthetic, but how one starts to deal with what those parameters of realism are is part of what you are playing with. It is what Godard was playing with constantly.

## Why did Sundance decide to launch an
## online festival in 2001?

It's something for me that is a first step. It's an exploration of something that should be done and it has been absolutely the opposite of what people would expect. I don't know of another festival that is trying to do this with the same mentality. I certainly think there are a lot of festivals that have showcased Internet production, usually with a mixture of work that has used a distribution network. I'm suggesting that the Web is something different than that. I think that the aesthetic of online production is something that is going to influence independent production and already has.

I had decided I was wrong to think of the Web as simply being a substitute network, so I began thinking about how Web networking would serve as a new system of distribution for a range of works that are floundering in the theatrical marketplace. Just to clarify, our intention is for this to be an annual event, but we're not putting the festival online. We're doing an online festival. None of the films that are in the Sundance Film Festival will be in the online program. It is a completely different program. There was a separate submission process and the films submitted were a range of different work, including a lot of animated work and a fair amount of work that is interactive. We're not trying to do a retrospective of films that have been sold to a lot of the online Web sites. We're trying to look at new aesthetics, what Internet production is all about. To me, ultimately it's new, something that is innovative and again something I don't think we've seen yet. In choosing the pieces, we looked at everything we could find and looked for the most provocative and interesting ideas, ranging from less than an hour to a couple of minutes. The delivery system is still very difficult. We're trying to do what we can.

I can't tell you I'm overwhelmed by the quality of what is submitted, but I think it's interesting. Again, I am of the belief that the Web contains a range of different aesthetics that are going to be developed, and ones that we really have not seen. One of the problems that the Web companies have faced is trying to define what they mean when they talk about production. Those are the kinds of questions, the kind of aesthetic issues that I'd like the festival to showcase. If you want to be a company that is producing for the Web, one should actually showcase what those ranges are, really showcase the range of different kinds of work that can be done. It's not always about technology. It's a question of a certain kind of spirit, a certain kind of storytelling mode which I think can be very different. One could argue that the sprit of a *South Park* comes from an online production spirit and I think that's the kind of thing were going to see over the next couple of years.

### Why is there such a romantic spirit that infuses the filmmaking mythos?

There is that sense of the great American novel from fifty years ago; I think the great American film more or less replaced it and it reflects and embodies so much in us that is so personal and very social at the same time. I think that is one of the reasons that filmmaking has become such a sexy a kind of profession.

My son, who is ten years old, is enormously interested in media. He works with images on all sorts of levels—video, TV, film, computer imagery, Game Boy, Nintendo...but that makes him exactly the normal kid, not exceptional but someone who is growing up with a range of literary. It's not media literacy, per se; it's almost a literacy of the image. I used to call it filmic literacy, but it's broader than that. And I think kids have it from the time they are very young.

### Is there an oversaturation of that imagery?

I think it's almost the other way around. The people who are truly creative are given the possibility of taking and changing what they have been given so they can play against expectations.

They can play on the literacy or expectation that allows you to recognize the image as having a certain kind of a realistic connotation or almost a documentary connotation, and they can play with that. I don't think saturation has limited them. I think it has opened up the possibilities. I think a few years ago finances dictated the kind of image choices independents made. But now it's more about aesthetic choices and how modes of production can serve the image. Yes, we saw more experimentation in our submissions this year than last, but not nearly in the kinds of numbers that would convince you the digital revolution has arrived. Quite honestly, I'd love to see more experimentation happening on film, irrespective of what's happening on video.

**Do you feel that Sundance is one step ahead of our culture?**

I do think we're setting an agenda rather than reflecting one. I've think we've really tried to expand the possibility of what independent cinema is and I think we've really tried to stay one step ahead of the fray here, as much as we can. We're trying to showcase work that represents overall that spectrum of independent, cinema but I've never felt obligated to showcase films simply as examples. We showcase what we think is quality. Last year we had more films picked up than any other year since 1996. So you have an enormous number of films that have had their premieres at Sundance that are actually in the market that didn't go to a lot of other festivals.

**With so many festivals, so much competition to be "first," how do you hold on to your reputation as one of the world's premiere film festivals?**

One of things we try to do is to be part of the discovery. I'm not saying we don't have some specific launches in the festival, but a lot of what we are still doing is looking at brand new directors and brand new works. We're not a showcase for distributors interested in just launching something. Instead, Sundance is a combination of a festival and a market, and for that I have no apologies...it is a place where work can get sold—I have said that one of the nicest things you can do for a filmmaker is get him or her out of debt.

# PIERS HANDLING
## Director, Toronto International Film Festival

Piers Handling is the Director of the Toronto International Film Festival Group, which consists of the Toronto Film Festival, Cinematheque Ontario, Sprockets, The Film Circuit and The Film Reference Library. He has organized numerous programs and retrospectives over the past fifteen years for the Festival including major retrospectives of Canadian, Latin American, Italian, Polish, Portuguese and Hungarian cinema. Handling has also written extensively on Canadian cinema and has been published in numerous film journals.

After beginning life as a small upstart on the international circuit in 1976, the Toronto Film Festival is now considered one of the world's premiere film festivals, but has never lost its prime objective: to celebrate and promote the Canadian achievements in an international forum by bringing together local, national and international films, and introducing them to the world.

Along the way, they have established a reputation for showcasing indie films from around the globe. Amongst the notables: Poland's Agnieszka Holland with *Europa, Europa* (1990); UK's Antonia Bird's *Priest* (1994) and the USA's Todd Solondz's *Welcome to the Dollhouse* (1995), which also had its world premiere at the festival.

**What were these "25 by 25" DV film commissions about?**

We were looking for an idea to commemorate the 25th anniversary of the festival. We wanted to commission these shorts and get the filmmakers to concentrate on their festival memories and experiences but we realized when we limited it to Canadian filmmakers that there were a lot of international filmmakers who come here and I was looking for a way to involve them.

I went down to Los Angeles and lunched with Next Wave Film's Peter Broderick. We were chatting about this and that and Peter said that at his millennial New Year's Eve party all the guests had to either bring a film or were given a digital camera and told to make a film of the party. I thought that was a great idea. We honed the idea down to twenty-five hours to shoot, a few hours to edit, and the filmmaker would shoot his or her festival experiences. We'll offer it to visiting filmmakers. It's a way for them to be creative and to give our audiences an insight as to what it's like being a filmmaker at the festival...a "day in the life" if you will.

## When did you start using digital projectors?

We ran digital projectors here in 1999, for five features, but we didn't tell many people. We did it quietly on purpose. For one thing, we weren't sure what is was going to mean to our future. Right now we look at about 1500 films on tape, and that's a lot of features to look at. If we suddenly specified digital, we could've had another 1500 films and there was no way we could physically deal with that, even in the pre-selection process. We simply don't have the manpower to look at that much material.

## How does it change the festival?

I don't think it's really changed the festival that much, but we're obviously looking at more films shot on DV. It allowed us to show Bernard Rose's [*Immortal Beloved*] first DV feature *ivansXtacy*, which we wouldn't have been able to show otherwise as there is no print of the film. We wanted the option in the event that film-makers we had been dealing with in traditional formats decided to move into digital video. We wanted to show that, increasingly, this was going to be part of our future. We would be able to say, absolutely, we can show your film.

## Do you think digital video is going to create a new grammar of cinema?

I don't think so. The basic grammar of cinema has been defined for years. I think it's perfect for a certain group of filmmakers ready to free their imaginations.

## Certainly it has influenced the style.

If it's that jumpy, handheld video style that you're talking about, then yes. The music video over the past fifteen years has had an enormous impact on feature filmmaking in terms of the dura-tion of shots, in terms of what young kids expect to see on screen...the vibrancy of color and of movement. DV to some extent is an extension of the music video. For me there is an interesting crossover stylistically.

## Is it all about being about to make films for less money?

Partially, although I don't think Lars von Trier moved to DV just because of money. I think stylistically it has given them a degree of freedom and sense of play. The DV camera changes your whole relationship to the production process. I talked to Deborah Unger, who worked on Jonathan Noissiter's *Signs & Wonders*. She said that as an actor, it was rather difficult and disconcerting for her in a way to be in a DV shoot. In a flash, they'd take a scene that wasn't working inside and move it outside. You can go to a film shoot where DV is being used and you can't tell where the camera is. At a 35mm shoot there's that cluster around the camera—it's so big, so predominant. DV changes everything.

Also, early on, if you shot in DV people thought the sound or the image wouldn't be good, that it wouldn't look as professional. I think the Dogme filmmakers broke those taboos and completely reoriented many of us in the industry to look at the material.

*The Idiots, The Celebration,* even *TimeCode,* at the end of the day were all transferred to film and blown up to 35mm, but at some future time when all theaters are equipped digitally they won't even bother.

**What is it about those Dogme films that triggered such a wave?**

*The Celebration* is just so subversive and so well done, well made...a very smart script. That film could've been done on film, but it's also the one that worked the most. I think it's the family dynamics and how smart he is in terms of the relationships. *The Idiots* thumbed its nose the most at convention, and it was done on video....

**Despite the freedom, digital video has its own set of conventions.**

Yes and no. When you move a 35mm production into an office or a building there's a whole kind of paraphernalia that's just not there when you do it on DV. That frees up a filmmaker in terms of what they can do with the camera and their imaginations. You just have to look at the difference between *Sunday* and *Signs & Wonders* to see what it's done for Jonathan. It's very free, very open. When you look at a Bernard Rose film it feels much more like a traditional theatrical film, though there are certain moments that are more handheld. It feels like he did this film very cheaply, very quickly and almost without being noticed.

**The digital video aesthetic also dovetails with the wave of "authenticity" that currently seems to be an obsession in film.**

I think it's one of the key elements of digital video, certainly of the Dogme philosophy, which is—lets face it, basically a return to the 16mm practice in the late '50s, early '60s—the French New Wave. Release the camera, take it out of the studio, put it on people's shoulders, do absolutely anything, cut anyway you want to. It doesn't have to be continuity cutting. We can jump cut in the way that Godard freed the stylus with film with *Breathless*. I think in a funny way Dogme's revisiting that forty years later, saying there's something that we've lost. It's all become very slick, very studio bound, very glossy and very stultifying.

**Why is Godard still considered to be so important?**

He was one of the first to move in the direction of video, more so than anybody else. His world view is probably out of date right now, but cinema is fashion. I think it is the same with any artist. But this whole notion of being in fashion, of being contemporary, I find disturbing. For me, Godard is timeless and I think people will catch up to what he has done in the last fifteen years. There are some actors who are completely loyal to Godard. If he were to phone up tomorrow they'd be in the film even if they had no idea what the film was about...just for the experience of working with genius.

Obviously, it was disconcerting for actors to deal with Godard. He wouldn't tell them anything...there was no psychological motivation...they must have felt like puppets. That is very different than working with someone like Bergman. Actors *adored* him. Godard is a genius, but do his actors adore him? Probably not. It's a very different experience. Bergman is closer to theater, while Godard is closer to pure cinema...Godard has disappeared in the way that art cinema directors can disappear. I think my generation will always relish the fact that you have people like Mike Figgis and Wim Wenders around making work. No matter if some it's failed. They still see films as art, and perceive it as a form of personal expression.

Regarding their DV projects, *TimeCode* did better than anyone expected commercially. *Buena Vista Social Club* did incredibly well. As more major artists begin to move in that direction...people will as well. So much of their work is drawn from experimental film....

## Are you of the opinion that celluloid will be a dying medium?

I was a doubting Thomas until about two years ago. For those of us that have been brought up on film there is a richness, depth, acuity and color saturation that you'll never be able to get on digi-video, but many art forms have changed over the centuries.

Art moves with the time, and I think film will as well. Celluloid will die, but I'm not sure when. In another fifteen or twenty years everything will probably be digitally equipped. The quality will be so close to what we are used to that the new generation won't know the difference and it will become an archival medium.

## Have you noticed any other trends in films?

I would have to note that in films such as *American Beauty*, *julien don-key-boy* and *Celebration* that the dark underbelly of the family has certainly been one trend. It's hard to generalize—I see four, five hundred films a year. At the end of the day it's really the same. People dealing with romance, love, family relationships, the quotidian problems most of us confront.

## But what constitutes excellence in cinema?

The best film is the most imaginative. I got involved in cinema because of Godard. His films had an immense impact on me. I've always carried that notion in my head of somebody who is totally prepared to challenge every single rule, who doesn't abide by the rules of the game and is constantly asking questions. That's the cinema I search out. It's not necessarily the only cinema that I show here. I have broad, catholic tastes, but if somebody said to me you're going to have a film festival and you're going to invite ten to fifteen films, the kinds of films I would invite would be "high art" films—the new Iranian films, some of the most severe French films—it's the Antonionis and Wenders of this world, the Godards and Bressons, whom I admire the most.

I think it is the same for almost every director of a festival. You want to challenge or unsettle your audience, not reinforce beliefs that are already in place. When I saw my first Godard films they totally unsettled me. They forced me to ask so many questions about film, the medium, all my preconceptions about narrative. Here was someone saying, I'm going to challenge every single assumption you have in terms of what a film is...I will always have the softest part of my heart for filmmakers who are not trying to replicate Godard, but who are always asking questions—about image, about form, about using the grammar of cinema in innovative, different ways. Which is why, although he is not one of my favorite filmmakers, I have great admiration for what Lars von Trier is doing.

**Someone called him the antichrist of celluloid.**

I'm not sure I really trust what he does, but I admire what he is doing, I really do.

**He does deconstruct cinema in a very challenging way.**

In the same way that Cassavetes did, and I admire his contribution to American independent cinema. He is one of the pioneers.

**Have the politics of cinema changed over the years?**

Enormously. I think there is a cynicism that has crept in. Generally speaking, films are made now to entertain. There are very few countries—Iran is one, China perhaps another—where film is used in a different way. It is used to reflect the culture, not to entertain in the traditional sense of the word. It is used to elucidate, educate, inform...the great ideal of the '60s was that cinema would change the world. I don't think anyone feels that way any longer. But perhaps they do in these countries where they are undergoing immense cultural shocks, if not actual revolution.

For those filmmakers, there is a real validity to what they're doing. They have an audience that looks to them to express their dreams in some kind of way. I'm always reminded of the Russian poets and how important poetry was in the Soviet Union. Those guys, like Yvestchencko, were like rock stars.

They had readers numbering in the millions, and when they published it was the collective dreams of the Soviet people that went into their poetry, something that couldn't be expressed in the official culture. Zhang Yimou in China is constantly running into problems, as are Abbas Kiarostami and Kandahar Mohsen Makhmalbaf in Iran. How many Western filmmakers are censored anymore? They have complete freedom but, I think, have lost a sense of what they want to talk about. The audience for serious work seems to have gone away. Viewers don't want to be challenged or reminded of their political and ideological failures.

**Do all you festival programmers get together and discuss the politics of filmmaking?**

Geoff Gilmore [Sundance] and Richard Peña [New York Film Festival] and I have been on panels together and I like them both enormously. We don't talk about the film selection process as we're going through it. We don't share information—it's very much every man for himself, or every festival. New York is close to Toronto in terms of dates, so we're basically looking at the same films, but when Geoff puts his program together, I don't worry because he is four or five months away from us. Obviously, there are those shared elements that all our lives consist of—the hassles, egos and politics. Richard's festival is part of Lincoln Center and showcases about twenty films per year. I don't think Richard could turn that festival into competition involving 200 films anymore than I could make Toronto a festival for twenty films.

**Do you take on higher profile, sometimes less "worthy" entries for the sake of the smaller films?**

That's totally the philosophy of festivals I would say. You need the glitz and glamour of major stars, major directors and major films to attract major attention and as a result and there is a smaller spillover to the smaller films. The Roger Eberts of this world go to the big gala but they also go and see a lot of the smaller films that there is a buzz about. Word travels at a film festival really quickly. Everyone's antennae are up, so it's important to have a balance of the two.

**Do festivals set the tone for the currency of cinema?**

I'd like to think that we have that impact. Festivals should be at the cutting edge. They aren't always, but I think that should be our role to go out and find new talent. That's not all we can do, but I think its one of the few key functions of the festival to show work by first time filmmakers...to really give them a chance. A lot of first-time filmmakers are taking chances that other filmmakers aren't.

There's a vibrancy, a freshness and daring that should be supported. Clearly, as they move into the industry they tend to become a little more conservative, and they don't need festivals in the same way. Festivals are the great marketing tool. They really level the playing field and attract an enormous amount of external attention. A filmmaker's career can literally be made in the course of a festival. It's a world where you can still come out of nowhere and by the end of the party be a very hot property.

# TODD MCCARTHY
## Senior Critic, *Variety*

Fanatical about films since he was a teen growing up in Evanston,
Illinois, Todd McCarthy knew that he wanted to study cinema
when he headed off to college at Stanford. He became the
critic for the Stanford Daily for four years, and, after college he authored 1975's *King of the B's* about the history of
B movies. Moving to Los Angeles, he worked for a couple of years for the King of the B's himself, producer
Roger Corman. He then became a second string
reporter for the *Hollywood Reporter*, as well as West Coast
editor for *Film Comment* before making his home at *Variety*
in the late '70s. Currently the magazine's chief film
critic, McCarthy is also the writer/co-director of the
wonderful 1992 documentary, *Visions of Light: The Art of
Cinematography*, which highlights the work of major cinemato-
graphic innovators, and the author of the 1997 book, *Howard
Hawks: The Grey Fox of Hollywood.*

### What do you think about the current state of film?

Let's start a little earlier. Way, way back, I wrote a big piece on
Hollywood cinema, before independent cinema really took off.
I would say this way the mid-'80s, for *Cahiers du Cinema*—they did
a special issue on American cinema—and my conclusion was, and
my opinion even now, is that the '80s was the worst decade for
American cinema.

### Why was that?

When I was asked at the end of the decade to come up with my ten
favorite films I couldn't even come up with ten that deserved to be
on such a list. A lot of people wrote that about film at the end of
the '90s but I didn't agree because due to independent cinema
and the fact that you had quite a few things happening on numerous fronts and quite a few really great films in the '90s, the decade
was much more interesting. It was right in the middle of the '80s
that I wrote that the situation is not going to improve until cheaper, portable, and—as I probably put it back then—video cameras
become available for people to shoot their own films, thus
enabling independent films to made more cheaply. So I was looking at this development at least fifteen years ago as a way out of the
logjam of absolute torpor and zero-creativity that was prevalent in

Hollywood at that time. I was not predisposed against this idea at all, and I think that finally, its time has come.

**Which brings us to Dogme 95.**

Exactly. My response to Dogme is that I smelled a rat at the very beginning. I maintain that to this day, and Danish friends of mine have told me, privately, that my suspicious were right. That more than anything else this is a publicity movement more than an artistic one. However, it has borne some interesting fruit. It's kind of exploded things. It's had more impact than anyone could've imagined at the time. When I came back that year and published the Dogme certificate in my column in *Variety*, I'm sure it was the first time anyone in Hollywood had ever heard about it.

I almost put it in as a joke. I thought it was the most interesting thing to write about after Cannes that year—at least to expose it to Hollywood, given the venue that I have here in town. I don't think anyone could've predicted what has come from it, but the fact that Vinterberg's film especially got such a good reaction and people like Spielberg and others were admiring it and meeting him and it won awards and so forth, really legitimized the whole thing and made people realize, hey, there's another way we can shoot. Hence, it's had a very interesting effect. I think you see in *Traffic* and in other films that have had major success that it's shaken these up a little bit, loosened things up stylistically, and now a lot more things are acceptable to people. So that to me, is the benefit. But I still think, at its very deep origins it was a publicity thing. If we can't get publicity one way we'll get it another. It was a very interesting aesthetic way of attracting attention to an extremely small film industry in a small European country.

**To platform such a stripped down form of
filmmaking in such a baroque venue was a
brilliant idea.**

Absolutely. I've heard stories about these guys sitting around being totally stoned coming up with these outrageous ideas, and now people swallow them. But they swallowed them because at its essence there is some value and validity to it. It opens up filmmaking, stimulates things a bit. And *The Celebration* was pretty good up until the big climatic denunciation scene where the son is calling on his father and exposing the whole situation there. I thought the visuals were completely inappropriate to what was going on in the final section. I thought they did not serve the story. It was way too much all over the place, not properly focused. It really fell apart directorially in that last part, but I was pretty much with it up until then. So I am more guarded in my opinion of *Celebration* than most people are. To me the DV was as distracting in that film as it was interesting. There were a lot of set ups in that film that he never would've done with a regular camera, and I thought it was a fair amount of jerking around in that film. I did think Dogme 95 it would be more of a fad than it's been. Everything has its day then something new comes along, so we'll see.

**Many of its aesthetics are being taken very seriously.**

It's just the aesthetic and the approach, the fact that it can me done cheaply and at its best it can have an invigorating effect on things. Whether you adhere to the rules or not—and how many have there been? Fifteen, eighteen Dogme films? It doesn't matter. The whole notion of shooting in this rough style and the fact that it's transferable to 35mm and can be projected and the fact that people aren't really bothered by it, that they're willing to accept it if they like what is going on in the film—that is all that matters. No one is sitting there with a checklist, keeping track of whether you have followed every single rule. That's not an issue.

**So you would agree that it has had a very strong ripple effect?**

Yes, but it became apparent to me seeing films at Sundance—and I've seen numerous digitally shot features—but seeing a bunch of them at Sundance this year, what I don't like about this finally hit me. It's the fact that this kind of quick, from-the-hip shooting style has a tendency to be very random and arbitrary in the camera angles, compositions and the set ups, and that there isn't any lighting per se. When there isn't any lighting, you have a very reduced palette and fewer dramatic possibilities in your cinematography. Finally, what it boils down to is that there is no *mise en scene*. That's what really bothers me. Because at heart, what I most respond to in films is *mise en scene*, that there is a directorial approach, that thought goes into the shots and dramatic values are brought out of the shots. That there are lighting schemes, color schemes, cutting schemes, all the elements that go into an aesthetic for filmmaking.

I saw a film in competition at Sundance that made it hit home for me, [Henry Barrial's] *Some Body*. I thought I was going along with the film; I forced myself to stay just to see what was going on and finally there was one scene when the camera was in the right place and was expressive of the dramatic situation in the film. It made me realize that in no other shot was the camera in what I would consider to be the right place, in a place where it expressed anything.

**What did you like at Sundance that was shot on DV?**

Rick Linklater's *Tape* was as good as get gets for a film like that with three people in one room. It was one of my favorite films at Sundance. What I'm told is that Linklater didn't like the way it looked projected on video, and that he is very anxious to have it transferred to look better on film. Nonetheless, it worked tremendously well. I don't attribute that one way or the other to shooting on DV except maybe in the performances. It is a terrific film. I just don't think it being shot digitally was either here nor there.

One of the best films to me, directorially, was [Scott McGehee and David Siegel's] *The Deep End*. It is completely about *mise en scene* and style and approaching a genre from a different stylistic point of view. Seeing those two films back to back, it really hit home for me what I think is missing: In 95 percent of the digitally shot films there simply is not a strategic visual style which is in any way designed to amplify or support the content of the film. The style is just the same, is just arbitrary no matter what the subject matter is.

**Doesn't that have somewhat to do with the nature of DV imagery?**

It doesn't have to be. You can have a stylistically appropriate *mise en scene* when you're shooting on film or on digital video. It's not the stock that makes the difference. It's that you have this little camera and you can put it anywhere and you want to shoot fast and you just want to thrust the camera into the situation. If they start using it in a formal, more imaginative way, to affect and create an image rather than just pointing the camera it will certainly become more interesting. Roger Ebert was talking a while ago and said that the emotional temperatures of film and video are different and you can't quantify it exactly. There has been some intellectual probing of this possibility and I sort of feel that to be true. Film is a warmer medium and you tend to have a more emotional reaction to it.

Here is the other thing I worry about: that basically you're not going to get too many filmmakers who have any life experience beforehand. They are filming when they are thirteen years old, before they've done anything and they're just going to shoot, shoot, shoot. They'll think it's worth looking at just because they've turned on the camera. If you go back before cinema, the whole thing that novelists would tell is to go out and live ten years before you even think about writing. Think about Joseph Conrad and Ernest Hemingway. They had something to write about. Film becomes so inbred.

**So you feel that one of the problems with DV is that filmmakers are giving into its immediacy?**

Yes, and what is effective, obviously, is that you can be intimate with the actors, you can move quickly, maybe catch moments that wouldn't have been caught otherwise. But for what interests me in film, you're sacrificing way too much, and I don't think there is sufficient compensation. There can be shots where you hand-hold the camera and follow around and let the shots last a long time, but they tend not to. I don't know whether that's a factor, whether it comes from shooting in digital or whether it's a parallel development of the very fast cutting style coming from MTV. It might be both.

Ernst Lubistch made this famous comment seventy or eighty years ago, that theoretically the camera can be in an infinite number of places shooting a scene, but in fact there is really only one right place for the camera in any given scene. If you really think about it, it's absolutely true and a really good director knows it. That's been almost completely lost in this digital shooting style.

**Some filmmakers say that after all this rapid-fire imagery what they long for are films with extremely long shots and periods with long, long silences...**

I can sympathize with that.

**Even though so many of the older films are
readily available, do you feel that craft in film
is being ignored?**

Paradoxically the work of older filmmakers is more available than it's ever been, yet people seem to be less intent upon it. I made a point of meeting as many of the old directors as I could.

When I was at the Stanford paper I made a point of meeting George Roy Hill, Sydney Pollack, Otto Preminger and Arthur Penn. Later on, when I came to Los Angeles, I knew Jean Renoir extremely well. I took movies up to show him every Sunday, early Chaplin, Stroheim, Visconti's later films and Buñuel's. He had known Orson Welles really well but he had only seen *Citizen Kane*. I met him through Truffaut, because I distributed two of his films when I worked for Corman. We picked up *Adele H.* and *Small Change*; it was only because I spoke French that Truffaut was comfortable with me.

He came to Los Angeles a lot to see Renoir, take his vacations. His daughter went to Berkeley, so through him I met Renoir and started spending every Saturday at Renoir's house. It was the highlight of my life. I made a point of meeting Fritz Lang. When I got here it was just the last possible moment that you could meet these people. I never met Sternberg, John Ford or Groucho Marx, but Raoul Walsh, Howard Hawks and Sam Fuller became close friends. I made a point of it. I so much revere what they do, and a lot of these guys didn't see that many young people. I didn't realize it at the time. It was probably fun for them too. I'm just sorry for the ones I missed...but my generation, the film buff generation of the '60s and the '70s, was really into the past and discovering the old directors and keeping them alive.

Now it is infinitely easier to access film history through Turner Classic Movies, AMC and your video store. Oddly enough, the current generation has complete access to the whole history of cinema, combined with an apparent lack of interest for it.

**They keep saying that American film culture has
swallowed the world marketplace and that
oppressed countries like China are the one
making films with true content.**

I think it's easy to overrate that. In regards to America, sure the world's getting smaller all the time. Different influences exert themselves in many different directions. Conversely, the French New Wave had a huge influence on the American New Wave directors of the '60s.

## Should the better film directors be film buffs?

No, there are no requirements at all. In America, it tends to be like that. You can be a complete naïf about it. A lot of the great directors—Welles and others -didn't go to many movies because they didn't want their minds clogged up with how other people approached things because they already had such strong approaches of their own. I don't think it's necessary to become a film buff to make films, because most of your references will be film. I'd just rather see a film by somebody who knows something about something else.

## If young filmmakers are disregarding film history to some extent, they do seem to be quoting Godard and Cassavetes quite a lot these days. Why is that?

In America it was Cassavetes, in France it was mainly other people, but Godard was in the forefront with *Breathless*—shooting in a new way, on the run, off the cuff, handheld camera on the streets, very little lighting—that kind of thing. The current equivalent of that is digital shooting. Godard, though, had very rich imagery for the most part. He had a few rougher looking black-and-white films, but his color films tended to be extremely lush.

## What is the positive fall-out of this modern, off-the-cuff filmmaking approach?

It's shaken things up a bit, and it's also opened things up. It does make it easier to shoot a film, but the problem with film being easier to shoot is, now anyone can do it...and 98 percent of the people who do aren't going to be that good, so you'll have to sit through a lot more bad films. On the other hand, it could result in a handful of very exciting films that we wouldn't have had otherwise, as the system per se is not conducive to really interesting work.

## Where can one look for the next wave of filmmakers?

I would guess that the Internet would be a place for that. You can potentially reach millions...people like its dangerous subterranean reputation...so that kind of thing is always possible.

**As DV becomes less counterculture and more
mainstream, how can you create something without being swallowed up into the marketplace?**

> Anything that smells even faintly of possible profits will be
> noticed by commercial interests and co-opted more quickly than
> ever before. Probably the only way to stand apart is by con-
> sciously resisting it, to be so marginal, radical, or outrageous
> that it can't be easily digested by the consumer culture.

**Do you feel that the film business has changing
to some degree because of DV filmmaking?**

> When I first came here fifteen, twenty years ago, the big question
> from young people was, "How do I break into the film indus-
> try?" It seemed like a fortress with big walls around it. The
> thinking was skewed to, "How do I get over the wall or jump over
> the gate...how to make the right contacts to get inside...?" That
> notion of inside doesn't exist as strongly anymore because you
> can go out and do it yourself with this technology. It's much
> more an open game.

**Isn't it also being perceived as a way for
producers to churn out cheap films?**

> That could happen, but it doesn't seem very producer driven....
> I think a lot of directors want to try DV. If the project is appro-
> priate to it and you can't get it done any other way, that's fine
> also. I just say there is no reason to apply this so-called visual
> "style" to every subject matter. The visual style for any film, no
> matter what medium it's shot in, should be dictated by the story
> and what the director is trying to achieve in telling the story.

**As the market becomes more "open" and the
technology advances, isn't there some question
about how the film themselves will become more
controlled?**

> You are talking about two different things. One is how a film gets
> made, the other is how the dissemination of films is controlled.
> Television, for instance, went from three networks to over a
> hundred channels. It's become infinitely more diverse. People
> aren't going to sit still for "control." Sure, if there is a big film
> opening on five thousand screens and it is being disseminated
> from one central transmission terminal that's been specially
> coded to deliver the film, that's one type of experience, but that
> doesn't mean it is going to be your only choice. If people don't

like that, there are infinite possibilities on TV, the Internet, and so on and so forth. There is no danger of being limited to only one experience.

## Do you think the content will become more diffused?

There's a real problem in that when you have the access, just because you point the camera and shoot something doesn't mean it's worth looking at. In the end I think it will once again emphasize the importance of writing, structure, and all sorts of things that might be considered old fashioned or stuffy. That's what people respond to—stories, characters—all the usual things that have endured for centuries. But anything goes now, in a certain way, and if digital video projection triumphs and carries the day then things will certainly become less interesting. I don't like the fact that the digital victory is considered almost a *fait accompli* even before the battle has been fought. There is this worldwide financial imperative that we must switch to video.

## If that's true, will celluloid go the way of vinyl records?

Probably, eventually. But hopefully not while I'm still alive....

"**At its apex** in the 1940s and '50s with Alec Guinness films like *The Lavender Hill Mob*, *Kind Heart and Coronets* and *The Ladykillers*, but little used since the '60s, Ealing Studios is about to be revived. The West London studios were recently bought for £10m by a consortium comprising Fragile Films (the company that produced the Spice Girls' *Spiceworld*), the property developers Manhattan Loft Company and The Idea Factory, a San Francisco digital development company. The consortium plans a digital production arm at Ealing, and plans to create films for Internet broadcast alongside more traditional fare. ❖ The partners say they will pump £20m into the studios and produce twenty films over the next five years. The first two will shoot shortly. *Lucky Break*, written by Stephen Fry, and directed by Peter Cattaneo (*The Full Monty*) is about prison inmates who stage a musical in order to mount an escape. It will be released next year with the credit 'Made at Ealing Studios.' The second film is Mel Smith's *High Heels and Low Lives*, written by Kim Fuller (who has the dubious distinction of being the writer behind *Spiceworld*)."

**EALING STUDIOS**, London

# CRITICAL REVIEWS

## DEEP FOCUS:
## AT CANNES '98, DOGMA 95 HAS ITS DAY
### BY TODD MCCARTHY, DAILY VARIETY CHIEF FILM CRITIC
### (MAY 1998)

Among the footnotes to the 1998 Cannes Film Festival was the appearance in the competition of two films shot under an artistic credo called Dogma 95.

The manifesto, which has but two signatories, Danish directors Lars von Trier (*The Idiots*) and Thomas Vinterberg (*The Celebration*), caused quite a bit of talk thanks to its "Vow of Chastity," a set of 10 quite stringent rules under which a Dogma 95 film must be made.

The "Vow," incidentally, has absolutely nothing to do with sexual abstinence—*The Idiots* contains gobs of nudity and an orgy that includes hardcore sex. Its intentions are strictly in the cause of aesthetic purity, a discipline with which to fight the "technological storm" that has swept over motion pictures, "of which the result is the elevation of cosmetics to God. By using new technology anyone at any time can wash the last grains of truth away in the deadly embrace of sensation. The illusions are everything the movie can hide behind."

The Dogma 95 rules, slightly abridged, run as follows:

1. Shooting must be done on location.
2. The sound must never be produced apart from the images or vice versa.
3. The camera must be handheld. Any movement or immobility attainable in the hand is permitted.
4. The film must be in color. Special lighting is not acceptable.
5. Optical work and filters are forbidden.
6. The film must not contain superficial action. (Murders, weapons, etc. must not occur.)
7. Temporal and geographical alienation are forbidden. (That is to say, the film takes place in the here and now.)
8. Genre movies are not acceptable.
9. The film format must be Academy 35mm.
10. The director must not be credited.

The aim of all these mandates, per von Trier, was to "cast off the burdens" and "escape from rigidity," to "regain lost innocence" in the way films are made. On another level, he said, "the Dogma rules emerged from a desire to submit to the authority and the rules I was never given in my humanistic, cultural-leftist upbringing; at another level they express the desire to make something quite simple."

In practice, however, what the Dogma dictates yielded are two films that look remarkably similar: *The Idiots* and *The Celebration* both bombard the viewer with grainy images, chaotic camera movements, unstable set-ups and willy-nilly jump-cutting. For a while, the approach can be energizing; it certainly enlivens what would otherwise be routine, hard-going exposition in *The Celebration*, for instance. But the same herky-jerky style proves inappropriate for the gravity of the film's third act, where a more grounded, less intrusive camera would have allowed the power of the climax to come through with considerably more force.

Already a cliché, more a publicity stunt than a style (von Trier himself ignored several of the rules in the non-Dogma *Breaking the Waves*, filming in widescreen and giving himself one of the most prominent screen credits in memory), Dogma 95 received its fifteen minutes of fame in Cannes this year and is very unlikely to enlist many more subscribers (especially in Hollywood, where the prohibition on a director's credit alone will be enough to discourage any interest).

But another Dogma emerged at Cannes this year as well, one not yet codified officially but which has a lot to do with what it takes this season to be considered edgy and au courant.

According to what was onscreen this year, the following are the Dogma 98 rules for international art cinema:

*1. Include as much full-frontal male nudity as possible.*

After years of coyly turning actors around or framing them just so in nude scenes, the bread is out of the basket, so to speak, as filmmakers seem to be going out of their way to emphasize what was so long forbidden. In a mere Cannes sampling, male members were featured prominently in the aforementioned *The Idiots* (von Trier and U.S. distrib October are talking about using the old skin magazine technique of blacking out the offending area of the hardcore scenes to gain an R rating), Patrice Chereau's *Those Who Love Me Can Take the Train* from France (Vincent Perez in the middle of a

sex change), John Maybury's Francis Bacon biopic *Love Is the Devil* from the U.K., Ana Kokkinos' Aussie gay/Greek drama *Head On*, Francois Ozon's *Sitcom* from France and Todd Haynes' *Velvet Goldmine*, with the ubiquitous Ewan McGregor.

*2. Depict a liberal supply of rough/unsatisfactory/abusive and/or paid sex.*

This goes for films across the board, gay and straight. In fact, I can only think of two or three films in Cannes in which a woman enjoyed evident sexual fulfillment, most notably Benoit Jacquot's *The School of Flesh*, with the wondrous Isabelle Huppert. Most of the films in category one fit into this section, as do Lodge Kerrigan's *Claire Dolan* (in which Katrin Cartlidge's prostitute never seems to be satisfied even by the men she desires), Hector Babenco's *Foolish Heart* (in which, as in many of the films, the man finishes his business in a matter of seconds), Hal Hartley's *Henry Fool* (ditto), *The Celebration*, Shohei Imamura's *Kanzo Sensei*, Erick Zonca's *The Dreamlife of Angels* and Alexi Guerman's *Khrustalyov, My Car!*, in which a man is defiled with a shovel.

*3. Put the spotlight on what is now regarded as the most taboo of crimes, pedophilia.*

Sex with children constitutes a major preoccupation in Todd Solondz's excellent U.S. indie *Happiness*, *The Celebration*, Claude Miller's *The Class Trip* from France, Victor Gaviria's *The Rose Seller* from Colombia, just among the films I saw. Apparently, the "Lolita" curse hasn't discouraged any number of international filmmakers from pushing fearlessly into this deeply disturbing area.

*Article reprinted courtesy of the author.*

# STRAIGHT TO FILM:
## CAN VIDEO CUT IT ON THE BIG SCREEN?
## THE PROS AND CONS OF TAPE TO FILM
## AND VIDEO-IZATION OF THE MOVIES.

BY GAVIN SMITH, *FILM COMMENT*
(JULY—AUGUST 1997)

"The great hope is that now with these little 8mm video recorders...one day some little girl in Ohio is going to be the new Mozart and make a wonderful movie," pontificates Francis Coppola in *Hearts of Darkness*, the 1991 documentary about the making of *Apocolypse Now*. Even as he spoke, American avant-garde film had admitted to its pantheon Sadie Benning—a teenager from Milwaukee who used a low-resolution Fisher-Price PixelVision videocamera to explore her inner world.

Echoing the domestication of video in the past dozen years—the assimilation of the VCR and the camcorder into daily life—mainstream cinema was quick to make room for video its visual vocabulary. Video surveillance, secondary characters with camcorders, and cutaways to camera-viewfinder POV's have become a reflective plot accessory/stylistic device, from *Get On the Bus* back to *Down and Out in Beverly Hills*. While the unsurpassed primary text remains David Cronenberg's *Videodrome*, Greater Hollywood waited until *sex, lies and videotape* to anoint the second coming of the home movie. Since then, cinema has embraced video as the "capturing device" of our age, surpassing the unfilled promise of Super-8 a generation earlier. If there is a hidden agenda in the movie promotion of the debatable idea of video's penetration and restructuring of all spheres of our lives, it may lie in its successful subordination of video to its own economic impera-

tives: video had gone from being an ancillary revenue stream to Hollywood's revenue base—it's not b.o. that counts now, it's units.

But remember the ad copy for Larry Cohen's *The Stuff*: "Are you eating it—or is it eating you?" While Hollywood exploited video's economic possibilities, video stage aesthetic coups d'état. Video's most profound implication for the movies is the demystification and annexation of control that the VCR represents. What was once overpowering and unstoppable now obeys the viewers's PAUSE, REVIEW and STOP controls. Sublimating its hostility, Hollywood now makes its blockbuster action/SPFX flicks for the VCR. The escalation of EPM (edits per minute) and the ever more frenetic, attenuated, and incoherent construction of spectacle—appreciable in the mere year separating *The Rock* and *Con Air*—seem designed to satisfy freeze-frame and slo-mo connoisseurship. Consolidating this aesthetic takeover, video technology has captured two key levers of the filmmaking process. Filmmakers have been directing from behind video assist monitors for nearly fifteen years now—even during shooting they're video spectators. And the switch to nonlinear digital editing has accelerated the postproduction process at the expense of considered editorial decision-making. More crucially, edit-intensive cutting—formerly a painstaking process not embarked on lightly—is now child's play, and indiscriminately deployed. More and more films appear to be cut by people trained at videogame consoles.

Yet for now video remains film's visual inferior: it cannot equal 35mm resolution, and in particular there are still problems with both onscreen and camera motion blur (known as strobing) that are inherited in the transfer from 30 frames-per-second to 24 frames-per-second. But film also has, for lack of a better term, a *moral* problem with video, which is admitted to movie territory mostly as an inferior, suspect Other. Certainly film's rapid surrender of the pornography sector to video in the early years of home-video's emergence conveniently tainted the upstart medium. In the movies, video is implicitly impure or impersonal at best; more usually, it connotes the sinister insidiousness of surveillance, the banality of TV or generic/estrangement/voyeurism/malevolence, as in *Lost Highway*.

"My love for you is impossible to show on screen," affirms French writer-director Alain Cavalier to his lover in *La Rencontre*, a highlight of this year's San Francisco Film Festival. This unique film merges essay, diary and personal documentary in an attempt to disprove that observation—and its first act is to abandon film for video. Shot in Hi8, edited on video, and then transferred to 35mm, it's an album of intensely subjective images linked by voiceover observations, confidences, and exchanges between Cavalier and his unnamed lover. Rather than chronicle the development of the relationship, Cavalier attempts to capture the renewed awareness and sensory wonder that romantic involvement spurs—and the antisocial impulses it harbors

His method is rooted in the devoted scrutiny of a succession of still-life tableaux consisting of small, commonplace objects and details—a pebble, a leaf, a fish, a dead bird, a key, a dissolving aspirin, a pine cone—which constitute a private language or iconography. The view is not furnished with a translation, a way of decoding and extracting the personal associations that underwrite any image.

*La Rencontre* is visualized and structured around the denial and exclusion of the outside world and its replacement with a private realm of contemplation and privileged objects and spaces. Never fully onscreen, Cavalier and his lover exist as disembodied voices and fleeting physical fragments—hands, feet, etc. Yet even as it pursues the ineffable, *La Rencontre* voices doubts and reservations: "If people see [the film], it won't be ours anymore," the woman objects.

If this conceit never quite succumbs to its own preciousness, it's because Cavalier pursues it with absolute commitment and discipline; its rigor redeems it from self-indulgence. And as the originating format, video reinforces this: Cavalier uses its cooler, more impersonal affect to counter the potential smothering intimism of the material. The video image's weightless translucence and discreet inertia, and the camcorder's self-effacing *camera-style* simplicity fit naturally with the ascetic-yet-lyrical minimalism of Cavalier's compositions. Even the camcorder's (at times visibly fluctuating) auto exposure evokes the evanescence of instability of emotional ebb and flow. Where mainstream narrative film implicitly views video as a debased medium, in *La Rencontre* it has never seemed as pure.

The standard process for transferring video to film is kinescope (telecine is the reverse). Now quite common in visually functional documentary, most notably *Hoop Dreams* and *Visions of Light*, it has also been successful in experimental work like Derek Jarman's staggering, trailblazing 1987 *The Last of England* (which transferred Super-8 to one-inch video for editing and treatment and then back onto 35mm) and Michael Almereyda's delightful PixelVision featurette *Another Girl Another Planet*. Recently there has been a mini-wave of tape-to-film features, ranging from the inept, self-satisfied would-be cult digital video film *Love God* to Rob Nilsson's brooding, visually striking, post-Cassavetes pool hall redemption drama *Chalk*. Underscoring the fact that video isn't a substitute for film, *La Rencontre* is transferred through rephotography—a less orthodox, more experimental method. In rephotography, the edited video is played on a TV monitor and reframed and filmed directly off the screen in 35mm at 30 fps. The most notable recent example is German filmmaker Fred Keleman's Hi8 long-take doomfest, *Fate,* a neo-direct cinema study in cultural dispossession and urban abjection.

Where kinescoped video's, "clean," transparent transfer would make the fundamental irreconcilability of the chemistry of film and the electronics of video, rephotographed video by contract accentuates their differences, stressing the visible pictorial surface of TV screen with its kinetic pixel texture. (Again, video's fixed pixel grid is antithetical to film's unfixed grain field.) By rephotographing *La Rencontre*, Cavalier affirms that what we are watching is more that TV yet less than film—an intermediate form with its own aesthetic autonomy.

Lars von Trier's enigmatic ventures into transmedia processing seem motivated more by an interest in pure texture experimentation. His 1988 made-for-TV *Medea* (or should is be called *Media?*) was shot and edited on video, rephotographed off a TV monitor on 16mm and then transferred back to video again (the completed work only exists in tape format). The resultant grainy, washed out texture degradation suggests an archaic, pre-technological visual idiom. Conversely, *Breaking the Waves* film/video fusion—35mm Panavision telecined to video for color desaturation, then kinescoped back to 35mm, acquiring video pixilation in the process—is tenuously explicable as hi-tech cinéma vérité.

If film tends to enlarge real life into a movie, does video by the same token reduced it TV? Can that reduction be overcome by tape-to-film upscaling? Does one medium subordinate the other? The merits of the work come into play here. Compare Shane Meadow's *Small Time*, an unassuming micro-budget English film shot on video, and Chris Marker's *Level Five* (also at SFIFF). *Small Time* is *Laws of Gravity* via Mike Leigh—a loose, idiosyncratic ensemble comedy set in Nottingham about a gang of petty thieves and their wives. Mixing desultory naturalism and sharply observed parody, this affection spoof of Nineties English Lad culture underline the gap between fantasies of criminality the mundanity of English life. Shot in an offhand, knockabout style, its low-budget pragmatism carries it "beyond" video's limits. By contrast, the much-anticipated *Level Five*, the latest addition to the secret history of modernity that is Marker's overarching project, is sketchy and riddled with redundancy—a problem in a work predicated on information overload. An interesting forty-minute essay is inflated to a monotonous near-two hours via an enervating narrative framework featuring a female videogame designer's hazily-defined Dantean cyberquest to make sense of a repressed history—namely the mass suicide of Japanese civilians on Okinawa prior to the invasion of U.S. forces. Memory is Marker's great subject, but this conjunction of fascinating WWI history, oppressive digital legerdemain, and increasingly tedious cyber protocol (computers are, after all, memory machines) is at once overwrought and half-baked. Perhaps entropy is Marker's point, but this time his vision is impoverished by and doesn't "transcend" the visual and conceptual compression of video and computer-generated imagery.

There's a certain subliminal optical tension or unease latent in video on film, as there is in digitally sourced film imagery—the soothing flicker of 24fps doesn't neutralize the hard, unyielding electronic glare of video. I'm not sure why some cases this remains dormant and others flare into eye-ache-inducing

malignancy as in *Level Five*. At the risk of retreating into superstition and essentialism: only film carries the imprint of the real, the filmed object, in its form. In film, light becomes chemistry; in video it becomes an electronic signal, an analog of the record object rather than direction impression of it. And where the absence of film is a comforting darkness, the absence of video is the snowstorm chaos known as "noise." With digital imagery it's even more removed; those dinosaurs consist of Os and Is in complex arrangements with no origin in external actuality to make its likeness faithful, to keep it honest, if you like. (Neil Young uses the same augment in favoring the vinyl record over the compact disc.) Perhaps that's why CGI feels so soulless and unsatisfying after the initial frisson of spectacle has passed—it's simulation born in a sensory void. Mathematics and music are close kin, the but math of digital seems light years from Mozart.

*Article reprinted courtesy of the author.*

# CINEMA PURITÉ
## BY ANNE THOMPSON, *PREMIERE* MAGAZINE (AUGUST 2000)

Cannes audiences are usually a pretty tough crowd (their enthusiasm for slow-paced Iranian epics notwithstanding). But this year many of the 2,400 sleep deprived journalists and critics were reduced to tears at the first screening of Lars von Trier's *Dancer in the Dark*, a relentless musical tragedy about a blind American immigrant (Icelandic singer Björk) who will do anything to save her child's sight. The film, which went on to win the Palme d'Or and a Best Actress award for Björk, divided viewers sharply. Depending on whom you talked to, it was either amateurishly acted and crudely directed or a haunting work of visionary cinema. But even those who judged it harshly felt its emotional power.

In some ways *Dancer in the Dark* is a throwback to old Hollywood. The story line features the kind of unembarrassed melodrama we haven't much seen on the screen since the days of Douglas Sirk movies like *Written on the Wind*. And in dreamlike interludes, Björk and other characters suddenly burst into song with all the logic of '50s musicals. Yet von Trier's film is most stunning for the ways it rejects almost everything we take for granted in Hollywood movies: shot on digital video instead of film, it has a naturalistic look as gritty as the lives of the factory workers it portrays. The lack of additional lighting or re-recorded sound give many scenes the rough, imperfect feel of a documentary. Even the musical numbers have an unpolished immediacy—instead of being patched together from take after take, they play out in real time, the action captured by as many as 100 video cameras. And in the lead role, Björk gives an utterly unglamorous performance as raw as real life. "Björk is very special," her costar Catherine Deneuve said at Cannes. "She cannot really act—she can just be."

After two decades in which mainstream movies have often been defined by massive budgets, high-tech special effects, superstar performances and research-tested story lines, audiences and filmmakers are craving a return to authenticity. *Dancer in the Dark* was just one of several offerings at Cannes that were filmed more or less under the stringent back-to-basics code of the so-called Dogme film movement that von Trier himself helped start. And there was much talk at the festival about the growing "Dogme influence." But the back-to-basics movement in film is far broader than one would guess from the short list of films explicitly labeled as Dogme projects and has been going on much longer.

In movies as thematically diverse as Mike Leigh's *Secrets & Lies*, Larry Clark's *Kids*, Thomas Vinterberg's *The Celebration*, Eduardo Sanchez and Daniel Myrick's *The Blair Witch Project*, Kimberly Pierce's *Boys Don't Cry* and Mike Figgis' *TimeCode*, filmmakers have rejected Hollywood glamour, special effects and slick emotional manipulation. Instead, they are opting for a stripped-down, improvisational approach, one that is both psychologically raw and stylistically uncomplicated. In the 1960s, cutting-edge filmmakers brought refreshingly direct documentary techniques to what was dubbed *cinéma vérité*. The new movement toward simple, honest storytelling is today's answer to the superficiality of Hollywood. You could call it cinema purité.

Cinema purité confronts viewers with a kind of unfiltered reality, whether it's a drunken family-party revelation, a mother-and-child reunion, the fear of an unknown attacker in the dark, the breakdown of sexual identity, or an eavesdropper listening to her lover having sex. It plays with the cinematic conventions of time, point of view, format and performance. It's about looking at real life—in unflinching close-up. "I wanted to make a film for audiences who want to see human emotions from identifiable people of flesh and blood." So said Lars von Trier of his 1996 *Breaking the Waves*, a four-hankie love story starring a luminous Emily Watson, who was nominated for an Oscar®.

In March 1995, as a bit of a joke at the end of a drunken evening, the impish von Trier set out to "start a new wave," as he later admitted. He and director Thomas Vinterberg signed a document they called "The Vow of Chastity," promising to seek out only what is authentic in movies. Their Dogme films would use natural lighting and sound, real locations without imported props, and handheld cameras; they would ban special effects, shifts in time and place and "superficial action" involving murder and weaponry. "With Dogme they set a code that in many respects is the obverse of everything that is going on in commercial cinema," says Toronto Film Festival director Piers Handling.

Although *Breaking the Waves* foreshadowed certain aspects of Dogme, the movement would find purer expression in Vinterberg's *The Celebration* (which outgrossed *Titantic* in Denmark) and von Trier's own *The Idiots*. "It was half like a joke," says Kristian Levring, director of the Dogme film *The King Is Alive*. "We were all shocked at how big it became."

"A lot of filmmakers find it an exciting, fresh approach," says Bingham Ray, who backed *The Celebration* and *The Idiots* when he was co-president of October Films. "It allows them to create without worrying about technique." Harmony Korine, the 26-year-old American who wrote *Kids* and the wrote and directed *Gummo*, followed the movement's dictates on 1999's *julien donkey-boy*, which he improvised from a list of scenes and images, and spent $3,000 to obtain a "Dogme certificate" for his film. Actress Jennifer Jason Leigh, who stars in *The King Is Alive*, made up her mind to act in the next Dogme project she could find after seeing *The Celebration*. "It was visceral and shocking," she recalls. "It wasn't a contrived Hollywood story where you know the beginning, the middle and the end. It made me want to have that experience."

As fresh and galvanizing as they are, Dogme films have antecedents in a wide variety of moviemaking styles, from Italian neorealism and the French New Wave to the work of Americans John Cassavetes, Haskell Wexler and John Sayles. And perhaps Vinterberg and von Trier's manifesto didn't so much launch a movement as provide a handy label to a trend that was already under way. "It's the natural cycle of filmmaking," Handling says. "For the last 15 years U.S. films have been geared toward special effects and dumbing down. Filmmakers are rejecting the hidebound studio cinema of their elders in favor of freewheeling movies that are more personal, anticommercial. We haven't seen this kind of stylistic adventurousness and freedom for 30 years."

From the bracing rigor of such true Dogme films as *The Celebration* to the easygoing naturalism of such American independent films as *Ulee's Gold*, cinema purité movies share a commitment to immediacy and an aversion to all forms of film fakery. Though not all of these films share every one of these stylistic traits, here are a few of the hallmarks of the new cinema purité:

Ironically the new low-tech style of filmmaking is being made possible by a revolution in technology. Over the decades filmmakers have grown more adventurous as cameras got lighter and film stock more sensitive. Mike Figgis, blew up Super-16 film for 1995's *Leaving Las Vegas*, creating a look that, he says, "clearly defined the movie as not in the genre of the mainstream, high-gloss, anally retentive movie image Hollywood pushes out. "But advances in video technology—especially the latest generations of digital equipment—are breaking down barriers like never before. *The Celebration* was shot like a home movie with cameraman Anthony Dod Mantle wielding a

Sony PC7 video camera as a "family member." Actors were freed from worrying about where the lens was; Mantle's job was to be fly on the wall and find them, making instant aesthetic choices as he went. The results were electric and full of surprises. Similarly, the actors in *The Blair Witch Project* were their own cinematographers and the resulting faux documentary earned $140 million as much because of those rough edges as despite them. Jennifer Jason Leigh loved the freedom of working with three Sony mini-digital cameras and available light on *The King Is Alive*, the story of 11 bus passengers stranded in the Namibian desert. If the cast (which includes *Tumbleweed's* Janet McTeer) didn't like a scene, they'd do it again, until they got it right. "You just go and go and go," says Leigh, who plans to codirect (with actor Alan Cumming) a Dogme-inspired film. "There's no downtime in your trailer. You just start working. Nothing inhibits the actors. The cameras are so small, you're not aware of them at all." McTeer, who's now writing a movie with *King* director Levring, agrees. "It's about stripping off everything," she says.

Even big-budget studio films can find unexpected power through handheld techniques. The wrenching realism of *Saving Private Ryan*'s famous Omaha Beach sequence owes much of its impact to Steven Spielberg's decision to employ handheld World War II-era cameras for most of the shots.

For years directors have been forced to construct their movies using short takes from 12- to 15-minute magazines. And because of the expense of using more than one camera, most scenes are shot in countless repetitive segments—shooting first one actor, then the other—to create a conversation that will be pieced togeth-er in the editing room. The new technology has made it possible to shoot much longer takes, and from various points of view, which in turn gives the actors a freedom more akin to being onstage. "You get the joy of long takes and the intimacy of film," Jennifer Jason Leigh says. Mike Figgis fell in love with Super-16's 20-minute film magazines on *Leaving Las Vegas* and used the format again for last year's *Miss Julie*. Because of the lower cost of 16mm film, Figgis was able to shoot many scenes with two cameras, and often let the action run for the full 20 minutes. Knowing they have time means that actors "don't panic," he says. "They reach their stride about five minutes in; after ten minutes they're on some special energy, and they stay on it. The usual, incremental [movie] shooting style is the antithesis of good acting, like recording a 20-minute jazz solo in three-minute sections."

With his latest experiment, the $3.5 million *TimeCode*, Figgis carries his long-take approach to the extreme, shooting with Sony digital cameras, which can record for 93 uninterrupted minutes. Over two weeks, working on location with no script and 28 actors wearing digital watches, Figgis shot four synchronous 93-minute takes in the morning and spent the afternoon watching and discussing them with the cast. Changes were agreed upon and the next they would do it all over again. Since no input from studio executives was required, major shifts in character and story line were relatively easy to make. The film's ending was altered ten times before Figgis was satisfied, on November 19, 1999, the 15th day of shooting. "I never had that much freedom, to change my mind Tuesday based on what I'd done on Monday," Figgis says. Blown up to 35mm, the four synchronous quadrants unfold onscreen without interruption, with viewers' attention manipulated by sound.

In his harrowing drug drama *Requiem for a Dream*, which premiered this year at Cannes, Darren Aronofsky (*Pi*) also split the screen to follow different characters, and he attached small cameras to his actors to show a wide range of points of view. "I had four characters to deal with," he says. "How was I going to relay their different POV's? I really wanted to experiment and try a lot of new things."

To keep things real on his *cinéma vérité* masterwork, *Medium Cool*, Haskell Wexler threw his cast onto the perilous streets of Chicago during the riots outside the 1968 Democratic National Convention. Similarly, authentic, unprettified locations are a staple of today's cinema purité. For a subway-train scene in *Requiem for a Dream*, Aronofsky had to film on the sly, in the wee hours of the morning, with a tiny crew (a permit would have cost too much money). "Do you mind if we do it guerilla-style?" he remembers asking actress Ellen Burstyn. "Let's go!," she replied.

The Dogme collective hates manipulative Hollywood scores that telegraph every emotion. But a movie devoid of music can be an arid experience. In *The Celebration*, Vinterberg solved the problem by emphasizing songs the characters were singing and listening to. "If you cannot play on all the subtle emotions and amplify them by using background music, you have to trumpet them out through what is left, which means the cast," he says. "You don't have to have music to build a crescendo. The actors have to faint, puke or fight."

Lars von Trier obviously abandoned the no-music rule for *Dancer in the Dark*, which has musical numbers written and performed by Björk. "We used the idiosyncrasies of Björk's movements, which we learned to call Björkisms," choreographer Vincent Patterson (who also appears in the movie) said at Cannes, "because nobody in the world moves like Björk."

When the cast of a movie like *The Blair Witch Project* goes out to a real location and proceeds to improvise around a minimal set of directions, it is of course continuing a tradition marked by the work of such masters as Cassavetes, Robert Altman, and Jean-Luc Godard. Yet in the pursuit of authenticity, cinema purité can make unusual demands on actors. On *Dancer in the Dark*, Björk found the grim dimensions of her role emotionally devastating. At one point she walked off the production for four days. "She's not *acting* in this film," von Trier said at Cannes. "She's *feeling* everything, which was extremely hard on her and on everybody. It's like being with a dying person. And I worked like a hangman, in the sense that I was the one who dragged her there."

Director Mike Leigh has long fought the stuffy refinements of British acting technique, often putting his players through six months of improvisational rehearsals to refine his script. This method paid off on 1996's *Secrets & Lies*, with Oscar nominations for Leigh and stars Brenda Blethyn and Marianne Jean-Baptiste. And although last year's *Topsy-Turvy* (winner of two Oscars) was a classically beautiful period re-creation, Leigh's cast worked out the most minute details of their character's lives before filming began. "None of the actors knew anything their characters wouldn't know; they didn't know what else we'd shot," Leigh says. "We maintained this incredible sort of security and kept it all a secret.

So you get this organic spontaneous tension and truth."

Vinterberg went for a similar effect during the filming of *The Celebration*, by never telling the dinner extras about the nature of the family revelation to come—and then grabbing their shocked reactions.

While cinema purité projects may features such stars as Jennifer Jason Leigh and Catherine Deneuve, they are about everything but star power. The actors tend to be dressed down, deglamorized. (Leigh and costar Janet McTeer even picked their outfits out of their own suitcases every day.) And more often than not, the cast are virtual unknowns. If the *Blair Witch* trio had been played by recognizable actors, the movie would have been infinitely less convincing.

The same could be said of Hilary Swank's Oscar-winning turn in *Boys Don't Cry*, which stand in stark contrast to the way Julia Roberts plays the title character in *Eric Brockovich*. Both portrayals are effective, and both are based on research into the real-life people, but the filmmakers' intentions are very different. In many ways, Swank *became* Brandon Teena, successfully passing as a boy at home in Los Angeles (she told neighbors she was Hilary's brother, James, from Nebraska) and on the set. Roberts, on the other hand, did what she was paid $20 million to do: She used her star wattage (and cleavage) to entertain. "It was interesting because [the others on the set] didn't know me as Hilary; they just knew me as Brandon," Swank recalls. "Because I had already transformed for them."

Does anyone watching an Arnold Schwarzenegger movie every worry that he could possibly be in jeopardy? The eye-popping special effects, technological fakery, and catchphrase wisecracks common to Hollywood movies are part of an overall wink-wink, nudge-nudge approach that turns many films into kind of inside joke. The audience is complicit in knowing that nothing onscreen could possibly be real. In contrast, cinema purité is all about avoiding what's hip, ironic and jokey; these filmmakers are utterly serious about expressing real emotion and the consequences of human actions. When Jennifer Jason Leigh rolls around in the dunes during sex in *The King Is Alive*, you can almost feel the sand on her skin; when she retches with food poisoning, there's good reason to be afraid. Last year's Palme d'Or winner, *Rosetta*, rubbed audience's noses in the misery of a red-faced young woman trying to pull herself out of grinding poverty. When Hilary Swank's Brandon Teena breaks down in a police station after being raped, we feel she's a soul destroyed.

*Dancer in the Dark* has a goal not dissimilar to that of the old Hollywood melodrama: Make audiences cry. But von Trier and other Purité filmmakers are achieving that goal not through sawing violins or scenery-chewing, but through the immediate and intense ways audiences are drawn into the characters' lives. Despite so many advances in filmmaking technology, Peter Weir once told *Premiere*, "it's the close-up that remains the great invention of cinema." Now filmmakers, actors and audiences are rediscovering the unique power of film to communicate pure humanity. And not a moment too soon.

*Article reprinted courtesy of the author.*

# REFERENCES AND RESOURCES

## A VERY BRIEF TECHNICAL GLOSSARY

**Anamorphic** – A wide angled lens system that compresses picture information to fit into a small aspect ratio. To be properly viewed it must be uncompressed during projection using another anamorphic lens.

**Analog** – Signals created, measured and transmitted by variations in electronic frequencies.

**Digital Artifacts** – Undesirable, visual imperfections as a result of stray pixels.

**Aspect Ratio** – The relationship between the width and height of a picture. Determines a picture's shape. 35mm film is more rectangular than standard video.

1.33:1 – The aspect ratio of television, 16mm film and Super-35 film. Based on a screen measuring 4 units across by 3 units down.

1.66:1 – The aspect ratio of Super-16mm film.

1.78:1 – The aspect ratio of high-definition and digital television, based on screen measuring 16 units wide by 9 units tall.

1.85:1 – The aspect ratio of a 35mm film.

16:9 – The aspect ratio of high-definition and digital television, as expressed in horizontal by vertical units.

**Digital** – Information represented as computer data.

**Consumer DV cameras** – Topping at around $2,000, they are the least expensive and provide only the most basic image quality. As they have only a single video chip (CCD), it limits the overall image quality but allows them to capture images requiring minimal light. (*The Celebration*)

**Digital Video (DV)** – Video captured and reproduced as computer data.

**Frames per second (FPS)** – The number of film or video pictures taken or replayed per second.

24 fps – 24 frames per second. The rate at which motion picture film is photographed and projected in the U.S. and other countries.

24p – 24 frames per second progressive scan. A video format (as in the Sony PHD camera) that records video in a manner similar to a film camera.

25fps – 25 frames per second. The rate at which motion picture film is photographed and projected, and television images recorded and displayed in Europe and other countries.

30fps – 30 frames per second. The rate of images recorded and displayed by the NTSC television system used in the U.S. and other countries.

**Gigabytes (gigs)** – A measurement of computer data size. Roughly 1,000 megabytes of information.

**High Definition (HD) video cameras** – A wide screen, high-resolution video format featuring up to 1,080 of video. The high cost of using them makes them impractical for filmmakers making features on small budgets. (*Star Wars: Episode I - The Phantom Menace*)

**NTSC** (aka the National Television Standards Committee) – The American video standard based on 525 line images recorded and played at thirty frames per second.

**PAL** (aka Phase Alternation by Line) – The European video standard based on 625 lines recorded and played back at fifty frames per second.

**Pixel** – The minimum picture element from which video or computer images are created.

**"Prosumer" DV cameras** – Packing in more features and greater versatility, these cameras cost twice as much as the consumer models. They also deliver a higher image quality due their three video chips. (*The Idiots, The Cruise*)

**Time Code** – A system that assigns every frame of video a unique number that can be used for consistent and quick reference to that point.

# GOING GLOBAL: DV TRANSFER HOUSES

Although the debate continues, PAL is still considered to be far superior, to NTSC. It contains more lines of resolution (PAL has 625 versus NTSC 480), and at 25fps, the transfer yields a one-to-one frame correspondence.

There are also four main processes for tape to film transfer to consider: Although CRT is still the most common high-end system, there is also the Electron Beam Process, Kinescope and Laser. Each has their strong points and their weaknesses, based on what you are looking for in your image transfer and what your budget can manage.

Certain houses, such as Colour Film Services and Hokus Bogus, will only be able to handle PAL format film transfers, and costs can vary tremendously from house to house.

For a 35mm transfer: it can range from $190 per minute (Ringer Video Services) to $720 per minute (Sony Hi Def).

For a 16mm transfer: the cost can run from around $90 per minute (Ringer Video Services) to over $300 per minute (Filmout Xpress).

The good news is, many houses will do a ten second to two minute test, free of charge. As technology and rates are constantly changing with the times, it would be best to make contact ahead of time.

4MC (FOUR MEDIA COMPANY)
www.4mc.com
2820 W. Olive Avenue
Burbank CA 91505
Tel (818) 840 7144
*Four Little Girls, The Eyes of Tammy Faye*

CINERIC
www.cineric.com
630 Ninth Avenue
New York, NY 10036
Tel (212) 586 4822
Fax (212) 582 3744
*Mr. Death*

COLOUR FILM SERVICES
www.colourfilmservices.co.uk
10 Wadsworth Road
Perivale, Middlesex
UB6 7JX England
Tel +44 20 8998 2731
*The Filth and the Fury, The Last Resort*

DUART
www.duart.com
255 West 55th Street
New York City, NY 10019
Tel (212) 757 1580
Fax (212) 262 3381
*Series 7: The Contenders, Lisa Picard Is Famous*

EFILM
www.efilm.com
1146 North Las Palmas,
Hollywood, CA 90038
Tel (323) 463 7041
Fax (323) 465 7342
*The Anniversary Party, From the Earth to the Moon*

FILM CRAFT LAB
www.gracewild.com/filmcraft/index.html
23815 Industrial Park Drive
Farmington Hills, MI 48335
Tel (248) 474 3900
Fax (248) 474 1577
*The Farm*

FILMOUT XPRESS
www.filmout.com
1632 Flower Street
Glendale, CA 91201
Tel (818) 956 1185
Fax (818) 956 3298
*Sweet, Naked States*

GTC
www.gtc.fr
Tel +33 (01) 45 11 70 00
Tel +33 (01) 48 83 7756
*Such is Life, The Gleaners and I*

HOKUS BOGUS
www.hokusbogus.dk
Hokus Bogus ApS.,
Pilestræde 6-8,
DK-1112 Copenhagen K., Denmark
Tel +45 33 32 78 98
Fax +45 33 32 88 48
*Dancer in the Dark, The Idiots, The King
Is Alive, Kingdom 2, The Humiliated*

LUKKIEN DIGITAL STUDIOS
www.lukkein.com
Galvanistraat 4
6716 AE Ede, The Netherlands
also:
P.O. Box 466
6710 Bl. Ede, The Netherlands
Tel +31  318 698 000
Fax +31  318 698 099
*The Celebration*

RINGER VIDEO SERVICES
2408 West Olive Avenue
Burbank, CA 91506
Tel (818) 954 8621
Fax (818) 954 8431
*Hands On A Hardbody, Iron Ladies*

SONY HIGH-DEFINITION CENTER
www.sphdc.com
10202 West Washington Blvd.
Capra 209
Culver City, CA 90232
Tel (310) 244 7434
Fax (310) 244 3014
*Book of Life, Buena Vista Social Club,
The Cruise, Our Lady of the Assassins,
TimeCode*

SWISS EFFECTS
www.swisseffects.ch
Thurgauerstr. 40
CH-8050 Zurich
Tel +41 1 307 10 10
Fax ++41 1 307 10 19
Paris:  +33 (01) 6 07 10 42 82
New York: (212) 727 3695
*Bamboozled, Chuck & Buck, Center of
the World, julien donkey-boy,
Long Night's Journey into Day,
Saltmen of Tibet*

# RESOURCES AND WEBLINKS

## New Film School on the Block:
## USC School of Cinema—Television's Robert Zemeckis Center for Digital Arts
(www-cntv.usc.edu)

Standing alongside Robert Zemeckis, fellow alumnus George Lucas and Steven Spielberg have pitched in to fund this brand new, fully-digital training facility, which boasts the latest in non-linear production and post-production equipment, as well as production stages, and a 50-seat screening room. The first of its kind, it's designed to offer hands-on experience with the latest industry standard technology.

The Zemeckis Center also boasts an extensive array of visual effects equipment, an impressive digital editing laboratory with sixty of Avid's recently released Xpress DV systems, digital stages with motion control computers, CGI classrooms and digital compositing equipment. Among the other state-of-the-art features: non-linear digital shooting systems; a screening room with 16mm, 35mm and digital production capabilities and a THX sound system.

**DV FRIENDLY**
**PRODUCTION COMPANIES**
FINE LINE FEATURES
www.flf.com
*Dancer in the Dark, The Anniversary Party*

BLOW UP PICTURES
www.blowuppictures.com
*Chuck & Buck, Series 7: The Contenders*

GREENE STREET FILMS
www.greenestreetfilms.com
*The Chateau, Lisa Picard Is Famous*

INDIGENT
www.ifctv.com
*Chelsea Walls, Tape, Women in Film, Tadpole*

IFC
www.ifctv.com
*The King Is Alive, Waking Life*

NEXT WAVE FILMS
www.nextwavefilms.com
*Keep the River on Your Right, Maniac, Paper Chasers, Southern Comfort*

**DOGME 95 RELATED SITES**
www.elektropa.com
www.armybase.com
www.dancerinthedark.com
www.dogme95.dk
www.d-dag.dk

**PRODUCTION SUPPORT**
www.crewnet.com
www.zerocut.com
www.terran.com
www.avid.com
www.adobe.com
www.apple.com
www.digieffects.com
www.homemole.com
www.media100.com
www.pinnaclesys.com
www.digitalprojection.com
www.americanvideotape.com
www.indiebudgets.com

**CAMERAS**
www.canondv.com
www.jvc-america.com
www.panasonic.com
www.sel.sony.com
www.sharpusa.com

## CAMERAS (continued)
www.steadicam.com
www.dvdirect.com
www.jimmyib.com
www.steadytracker.com

## FILM INDUSTRY FILM FESTIVAL
## LINKS, PUBLICATIONS & RESOURCES
www.24framespersecond.com
www.4filmmakers.com
www.7dazemedia.com
www.afionline.org
www.afma.com
www.aint-it-cool-news.com
www.boxoff.com
www.cinematographer.com
www.cinematographyworld.com
www.cineweb.com
www.chapman-leonard.com
www.cnn.com
www.creativescreenwriting.com
www.dfilm.com
www.dga.org
www.dvfilmmaker.com
www.dvtonline.com
www.fadeinmag.com
www.filmfestivals.com
www.filmlinc.com
www.filmmag.com
www.filmsound.com
www.filmthreat.com
www.fipresci.org

www.hcdonline.com
www.hollywoodreporter.com
www.ifp.org
www.hollywood-911.com
www.indiewire.com
www.industrycentral.net
www.insidefilm.com
www.inzide.com/home.cfm
www.lcweb.loc.gov/copyright
www.marklitwak.com
www.milimeter.com
www.pkbaseline.com/screen/digest
www.premieremag.com
www.producers-source.com
www.resfest.com
www.samuelfrench.com
www.scenariomag.com
www.scriptsales.com
www.studiodepot.com/store
www.theknowledgeonline.com
www.variety.com
www.wga.org/manuals/registration.html
www.wordplayer.com
www.writerscomputer.com